SELF-EXPERIENCE

Kundalini Yoga Taught by Yogi Bhajan

Compiled and Illustrated by: Harijot Kaur Khalsa

Managing Editor: Ardas Kaur Khalsa

Yogi Bhajan Photo by: Satsimran Kaur

Additional Yoga Commentary: Gurucharan Singh Khalsa

Desktop Production: Khalsa Group Integrated Marketing

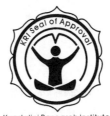

Kundalini Research Institute

Published by: Kundalini Research Institute Route 2, Box 4, Shady Lane,, Espanola, New Mexico 87532

Self Experience

Yoga means "union." It is the experience of Infinity in our own finite form. Kundalini Yoga offers us the discipline through which our self can experience our Self. It is a path that will lead us onward to find the bliss that is at the core of being human. It is the Divine Circle of life that the soul longs for the experience of the Creation through its human life and the human longs to merge again with Infinity. It is the Union of the self and the Self that we seek and that, paradoxically, can make us fully human.

Acknowledgement

The technology of Kundalini Yoga and White Tantric Yoga was brought to the West from India by the grace of the Siri Singh Sahib, Harbhajan Singh Khalsa Yogiji (Yogi Bhajan). The teachings in this manual are entirely his gift. We wish to gratefully acknowledge his gift and inspiration to serve our highest human potential. Any errors or omissions in this manual are entirely the fault of the editors and the illustrator and by no means reflect upon the perfection and comprehensiveness of the teachings.

*   *   *

The yoga sets in this manual are classes taught by Yogi Bhajan and are available on audio and video tapes. Although every effort has been made to communicate the technology of these classes accurately, nothing replaces the experience of doing Kundalini Yoga with the Master, Yogi Bhajan. Tapes of your favorite sets from this manual can be purchased through Golden Temple Enterprises, Box 13 Shady Lane, Espanola, New Mexico 87532.

About the Cover

The illustration on the cover was drawn by Yogi Bhajan. He explained, "This is called *longing*. The urge of the soul to merge. This is the only purpose of life."

INTRODUCTION

For Beginners...

If you are a beginning student of Kundalini Yoga, practicing for less than six months, or if you have been practicing without the aid of a certified 3HO Foundation teacher, please read this introduction before you begin to practice from this instruction manual.

Sadhana Guidelines

This manual has been prepared as a supplement and extension to <u>Sadhana Guidelines</u>, in which Yogi Bhajan, who brought the science of Kundalini Yoga to the West, explains yoga, meditation, and the Kundalini. Also important for beginners are the descriptions of the basics of Kundalini Yoga: asanas (postures), mudras (hand positions), bhandas (energy locks), and mantras (sound currents) explained by Gurucharan Singh Khalsa. For copies of this manual contact:
Ancient Healing Ways, P.O. Box 130, Espanola, NM 87532 , 1-800-359-2940.

The Teacher

Kundalini Yoga is a spiritual discipline which cannot be practiced without a teacher. However, it is not necessary for the teacher to be physically present when you practice. To establish a creative link with the Master of Kundalini Yoga, Yogi Bhajan, be sure to tune in to his energy flow using the Adi Mantra, "Ong Namo Guru Dev Namo."

Tuning In

Every Kundalini Yoga session begins with chanting the Adi Mantra: "Ong Namo Guru Dev Namo." By chanting it in proper form and consciousness, the student becomes open to the higher self, the source of all guidance, and accesses the protective link between himself or herself and the divine teacher.

How to recite the Adi Mantra:

Sit in a comfortable cross–legged position with the spine straight. Place the palms of the hands together as if in prayer, with the fingers pointing straight up, and then press the joints of the thumbs into the center of the chest, at the sternum. Inhale deeply. Focus your concentration at the third–eye point. As you exhale, chant the entire mantra in one breath. If your breath is not capable of this, take a quick sip of air through the mouth after "Ong Namo" and then chant the rest of the mantra, extending the sound as long as possible. The sound "Dev" is chanted a minor third higher than the other sounds of the mantra.

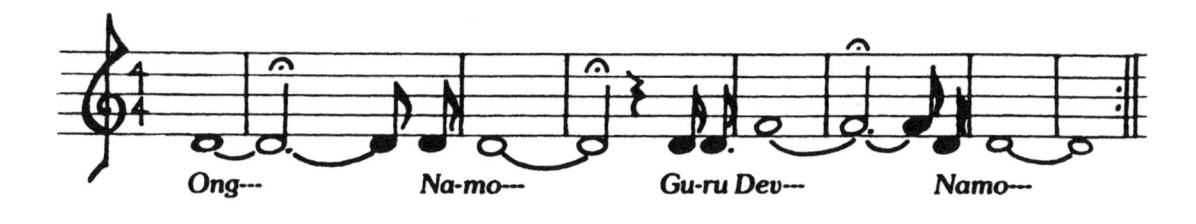

As you chant, vibrate the cranium with the sound to create a mild pressure at the third–eye point. Chant this mantra at least three times before beginning your Kundalini Yoga practice.

Pronunciation

The "O" sound in Ong is long, as in "go" and of short duration. The "ng" sound is long and produces a definite vibration on the roof of the mouth and the cranium. The first part of Namo, is short and rhymes with "hum." The "O", as in "go" is held longer. The first syllable of Guru is pronounced as in the word, "good." The second syllable rhymes with "true." The first syllable is short and the second one long. The word, Dev rhymes with "gave."

Definition

Ong is the infinite creative energy experienced in manifestation and activity. It is a variation of the cosmic syllable "Om" which is denotes God in His absolute or unmanifested state. God as Creator is called Ong.

Namo has the same root as the Sanskrit word Namaste which means reverent greetings. Namaste is a common greeting in India, accompanied by the palms pressed together at the chest or forehead. It implies bowing down. Together Ong Namo means "I call on the infinite creative consciousness," and opens you to the universal consciousness that guides all action.

Guru is the embodiment of the wisdom that one is seeking. The Guru is the giver of the technology. Dev means higher, subtle, or divine. It refers to the spiritual realms. Namo, in closing the mantra, reaffirms the humble reverence of the student. Taken together, Guru Dev Namo means, "I call on the divine wisdom," whereby you bow before your higher self to guide you in using the knowledge and energy given by the cosmic self.

Mental Focus

The following pages contain many wonderful techniques. To fully appreciate and receive the benefits of each one you will need mental focus. Unless you are directed to do otherwise, focus your concentration on the brow point, which is located between the eyebrows at the root of the nose. With your eyes closed, mentally locate this point by turning your eyes gently upwards and inwards. Remain aware of your breath, your body posture, your movements, and any mantra you may be using, even as you center your awareness at the third eye point.

Linking the Breath With a Mantra

A mantra is a sequence of sounds designed to direct the mind by their rhythmic repetition. To fully utilize the power of mantra, link the mantra with your breath cycle. A common mantra is "Sat Nam" (rhymes with "But Mom"). Sat Nam means "Truth is my identity." Mentally repeat "Sat" as you inhale, and "Nam" as you exhale. In this way you filter your thoughts so that each thought has a positive resolution. Mantra makes it easier to keep up during strenuous exercises and adds depth to the performance of even the simplest ones.

Pacing Yourself

Kundalini yoga exercises may involve rhythmic movement between two or more postures. Begin slowly, keeping a steady rhythm. Increase gradually, being careful not to strain. Usually the more you practice an exercise, the faster you can go. Just be sure that the spine has become warm and flexible before attempting rapid movements. It is important to be aware of your body and to be responsible for its well-being.

Concluding an Exercise

Unless otherwise stated, an exercise is concluded by inhaling and holding the breath briefly. While the breath is being held, apply the mulbandha or root lock, contracting the muscles around the sphincter, the sex organs, and the navel point. Then exhale and relax. This consolidates the effects of any exercise and circulates the energy to your higher centers. Do not hold the breath to the point of dizziness. If you start to feel dizzy or faint, immediately exhale and relax.

Relaxation Between Exercises

An important part of any exercise is the relaxation following it. Unless otherwise specified, you should allow one to three minutes of relaxation in Easy Pose or lying on the back in Corpse Pose after each exercise. The less experienced you are or the more strenuous the exercise, the longer the relaxation period should be. Some sets end with a period of "deep relaxation" which may extend from three to eleven minutes.

Music

Because of the emphasis on the integration of exercise, meditation, and rhythm in Kundalini Yoga, you will find specific music and mantra tapes used during the exercises. We recommend using the same tapes when you practice because they were chosen by Yogi Bhajan with precise effects in mind. If you don't have the specific tape used in a set, you may do the set without music or substitute other meditative music.

The Fingers

In the Yogic tradition each of the fingers relates to a different planetary energy. Through the positioning of these fingers in mudras one can either draw a specific energy into the body, project it out from the body, or combine it with the energies of other fingers to create a desired effect. The little finger is the Mercury finger and it channels communication. The ring finger is the Sun finger and it channels physical vitality. The middle finger is the Saturn finger and it channels emotion. The index finger finger is the Jupiter finger and it channels wisdom. The thumb represents one's ego or id.

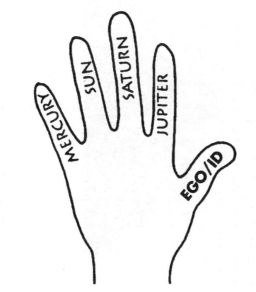

On Your Way...

The exercises in this manual are designed to be safe for most people provided the instructions are followed carefully. The benefits attributed to these exercises come from the centuries-old Yogic tradition. Results will vary due to physical differences and the correctness and frequency of practice. The publishers and authors disclaim all liability in connection with the use of the information in individual cases. As with all unsupervised exercise programs, your use of the instructions in this manual is taken at your own risk. If you have any doubts as to the suitability of the exercises, please consult a doctor.

We invite you to enjoy the practice of the Kundalini yoga techniques contained in the following pages. If you have any questions or concerns about your practice of Kundalini Yoga, please contact your local 3HO Foundation teaching center, listed in the yellow pages or contact the Kundalini Yogi Teachers' Association (IKYTA) at tel. 505-753-0423 or via Internet at Website: www.yogibhajan.com.

For information on courses and events world-wide, please contact the 3HO Events Office toll free number 888-346-2420.

"Experience and believe"
Yogi Bhajan

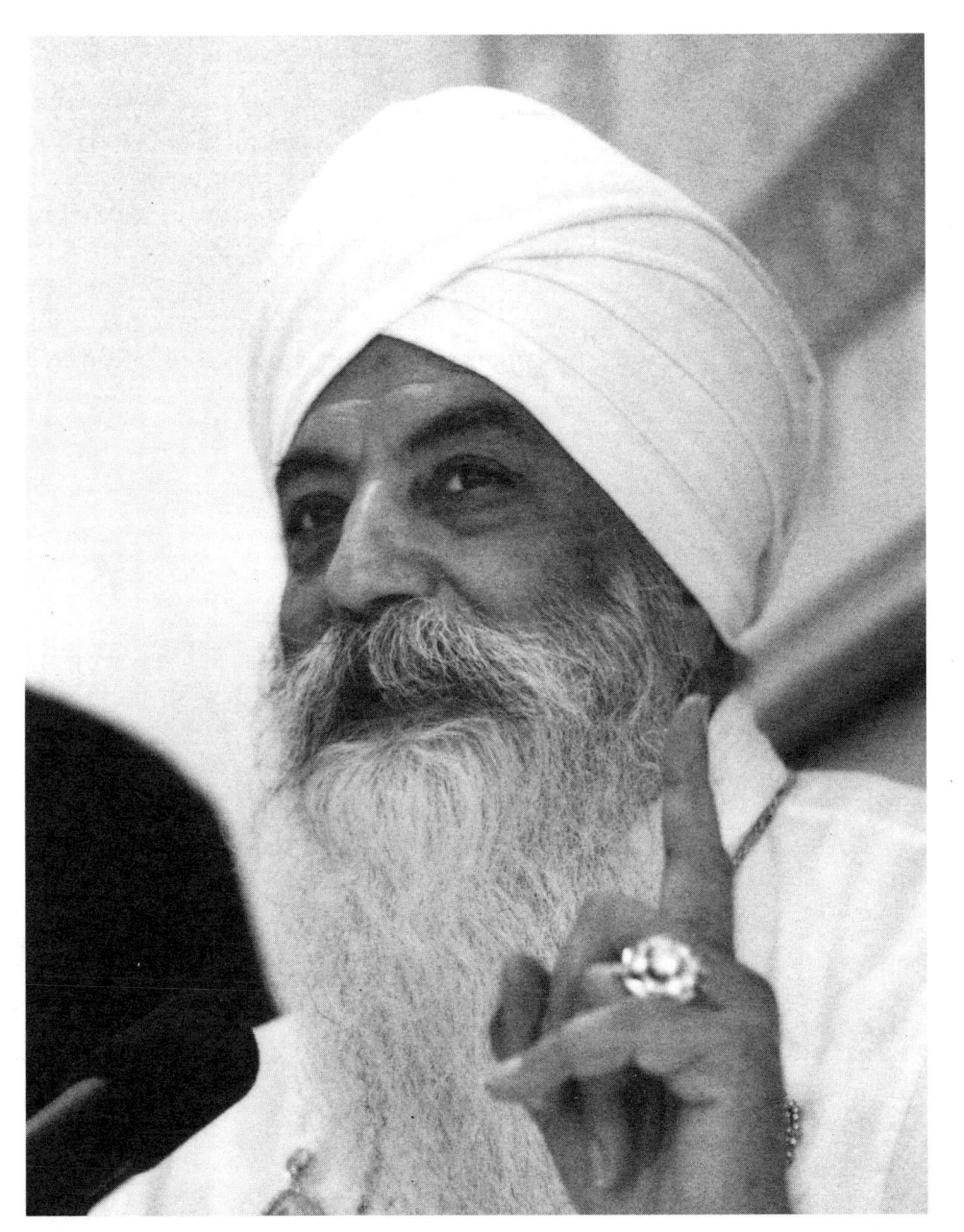

Table of Contents

Yoga Sets

Meditations

Music and Mantras

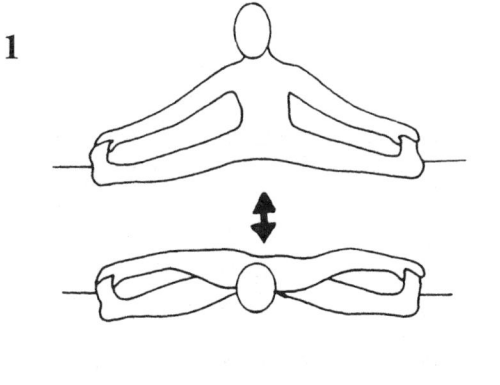

Adjustment of the Blood

June 14, 1984

1

1. Sit with your legs spread wide apart. Holding your toes, exhale and stretch down, bringing your forehead to the floor. Inhale and rise back up. Continue this up and down movement. 2 1/2 Minutes. Participate strongly. Bring your body into balance.

2. Lie on your back with your arms at your sides. Raise and lower your hips rapidly. 3 Minutes. This movement opens up the lower back and, if practiced properly, can prevent senility. Move quickly and powerfully.

3. Still lying on your back, bring your knees to your chest and lock your hands over the lower part of your ankles. Roll your body left and right. This side to side motion massages the lower back. 1 Minute.

4. Frog Pose: Squat down so your buttocks are on your heels. Your heels are off the ground and touching each other. Put your fingertips on the ground between your knees. Inhale through your nose and straighten your legs, keeping your fingertips on the ground. Exhale through the mouth and return to the squatting position. 52 Times.

5. Sitting in Easy Pose, bring your palms together in Prayer Mudra in front of your forehead, with your thumbs resting against the middle of your forehead. Close your eyes and breathe very slowly and deeply. 3 Minutes. This meditation can help to control high blood pressure and strengthen the metabolism.

"This set of exercises adjusts your blood circulation, because your blood must fully circulate to deliver the nutrients and energy of life to all of your cells." GCSK

"Kundalini Yoga is a very old science for realizing Reality within the realm of consciousness". YB

2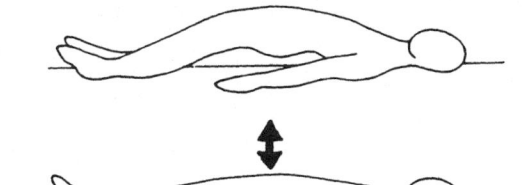

3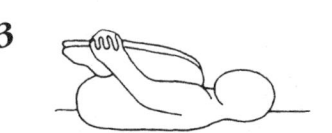

4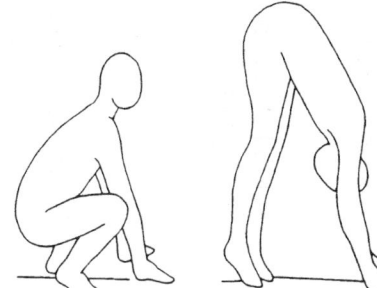

5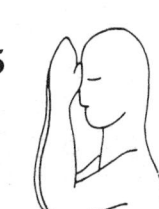

To Adjust the Heat in the Body for Improved Digestion and Weight Loss

August 31, 1995

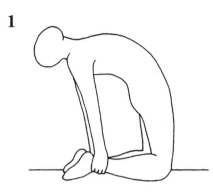

1. Camel Pose: from a sitting position on your heels, reach back and grab your ankles. Arch your body up, allowing the head to drop back. Hold this posture for 11 Minutes.

2. Rock Pose: sit on your heels with your hands on your knees. Keep the spine straight. Hold this position for 11 Minutes.

3. Baby Pose: from Rock Pose, lean forward until your forehead rests on the ground in front of your knees. Let your arms and hands, palms up, relax on the ground by your legs. Hold this position for 11 Minutes.

Begin by practicing each exercise for 1-3 Minutes. Work slowly and gradually up to the maximum practice time.

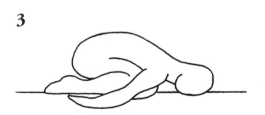

""The fire in you that lets you digest your food, also let's you digest the experience of the world. Each thought and sensation must be processed. With inner heat, everything is tasty and life is a joy". GCSK

"Live and let live and enjoy it. Experience it". YB

Awaken the Diaphragm

September 26, 1984

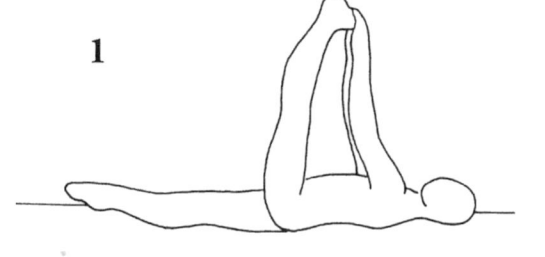

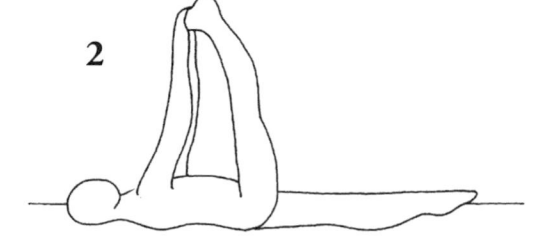

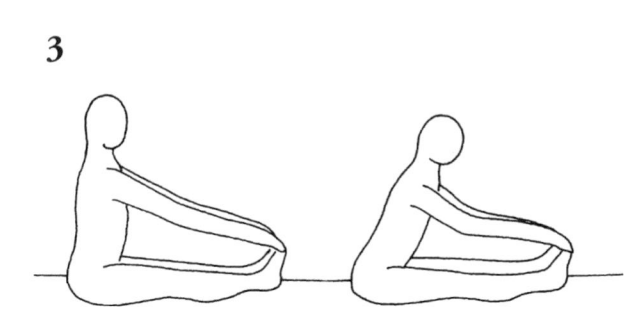

1. Left Charn Kamal Mudra: Lie flat on your back and raise your left leg up to ninety degrees. Reach up and grab the toes of your left foot with both hands. Keep both legs straight. Do not bend your knees. Chant "Har" rhythmically, continuously, and powerfully from your diaphragm. 6 Minutes.

2. Right Charn Kamal Mudra: Still lying on your back, raise your right leg to ninety degrees and continue to chant as in exercise one. Pump your diaphragm strongly as you create the sound "Har." 5 Minutes.

3. Kamal Prakash Mudra: Sit up and stretch your legs out straight in front of you. Grab your toes while keeping your spine straight. Move your torso down and up, bending from the hips, not from the neck or spine. Start out moving two to three inches and slowly and gradually bend forward more and more. Chant "Har" rhythmically and continuously from your diaphragm. 2 1/2 Minutes.

4. Lie down on your back and relax. 6 1/2 Minutes.

5. Shake your neck, shake your upper body, and then shake your whole body.

In exercises 1 and 2, you grasp the feet (Charn) and chant "Har" to stimulate your diaphragm and the lotus (Kamal) of the navel. Exercise 3 is a variation of Maha Mudra in which movement and chanting are employed to awaken the diaphragm. If you experience an inability to keep your legs straight or a lot of shaking in exercises one and two, it indicates that the organs below the diaphragm are not being properly served. The digestive system and the metabolism need work and fat is not being proportionately regulated. Your strength and stamina are about half of what they could be.

For a really powerful experience, do each of the exercises for 11 minutes. In about three days you'll experience "something you cannot explain or imagine." 11 minutes of exercise one and two can create a deep state of relaxation which cannot be reached by any other means.

"You have to conquer your laziness and ego. Insincere effort is a treachery with your own self, because you are not trying to reach an experience." YB

Conscious Re-birthing

January 29, 1986

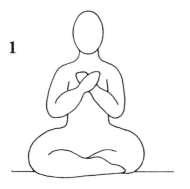

1

1. Sit in Easy Pose with a straight spine and cross your hands over your heart center, right over left. Open your mouth and breathe heavily through your throat. Close your eyes. You have to participate strongly. 7 Minutes.

2. Lie down in Baby Pose. Meditate on all the elementary pain you felt in your mother's womb and let it go.1 1/2 Minutes. For the final 3 Minutes, mentally re-experience the moment of your birth.

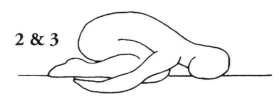

2 & 3

3. Stay in Baby Pose and go into a deep nap. 2 Minutes.
To finish: Inhale deeply and hold your breath for 1 Minute as you pump your navel. Feel beautiful and feel as if you have a tremendous amount of bright light in your head. Exhale and and inhale. Hold your breath for 15 seconds as you pump your navel. Relax.

4. Slowly rise up into a sitting position. Sing along with Singh Kaur's tape *Wahe Guru Jio.* Feel free and innocent and sing like a baby. 8 1/2 Minutes.

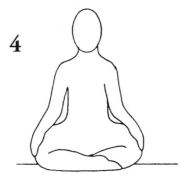

4

To finish: Inhale, hold your breath as long as you comfortably can, concentrating at the brow point. Bless yourself with the light of God. Use this light to rebuild and resurrect yourself. Exhale. Repeat this sequence two more times.

Sometimes during the first nine months of life, when we are in the womb of the mother, we pick up fears that become part of our personality. This conscious re-birthing kriya helps us to overcome these fears.

"You can never get rid of your fear, you can never get rid of your pain, doesn't matter what effort you make, until you have the guts to forgive yourself. Just forgive yourself." YB

4

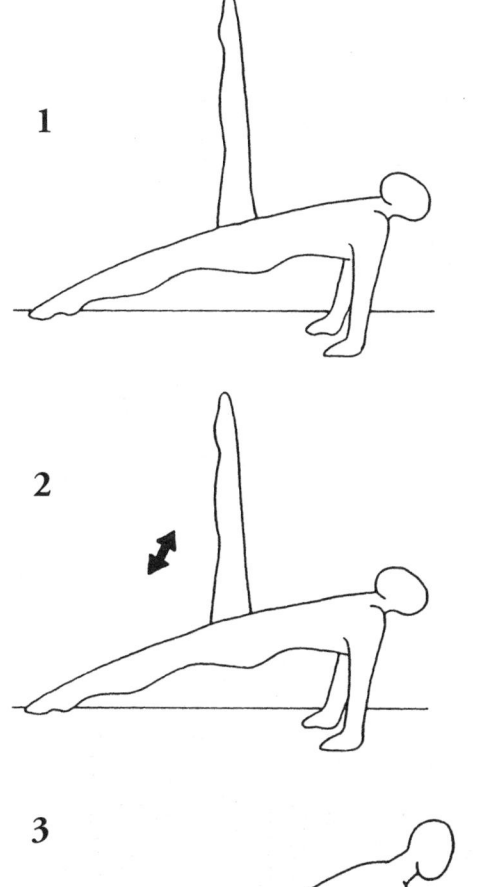

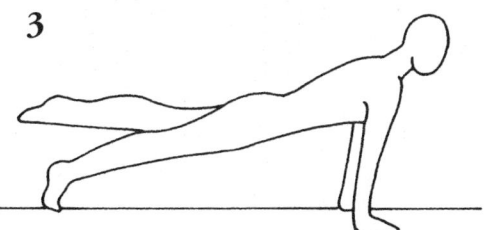

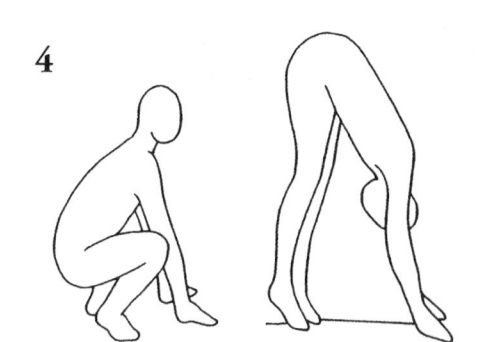

Adjust Your Rib Cage and Lower Spine to Develop Strength and Steadiness

June 21, 1984

1. Back Platform Pose. Your weight is resting on the palms of your hands and your heels. There is no bend in your knees and your back is straight. Lift the right leg up to 90 degrees, hold it in that position, and do Breath of Fire. 1 Minute. Change legs and lift your left leg up to 90 degrees. Hold it in that position. Breath of Fire. 30 Seconds. Begin alternate leg lifts with Breath of Fire. 1 1/2 Minutes. Powerful Breath of Fire, with this movement, can deeply cleanse the lungs.

2. Again do alternate leg lifts in Back Platform Pose. Lift each leg to 90 degrees with the knee straight, but not locked. Move rapidly. 3 Minutes. Continue leg lifts as you rhythmically chant SA-TA-NA-MA while you "kick the Heavens". 8 1/2 Minutes.

3. Front Platform Pose. Your body is straight with your weight resting on the palms of the hands and the tips of the toes. Do alternate leg lifts keeping your knees straight, but not locked. Lift your legs as high as you can. Musically chant SA-TA-NA-MA along with the movement. 3 Minutes.

4. Frog Pose. Chant "Humm, Dham, Har, Har" in time with the movement. When you move into the up position, chant "Humm Dham". As you move back down into the squatting position, chant "Har Har". 2 Minutes. A full cycle of chanting the mantra is approximately 3 seconds.

"When your navel is strong, and your spine is open and flexible, and your lungs are powerful, you have what you need to welcome challenge as a friend".
GCSK

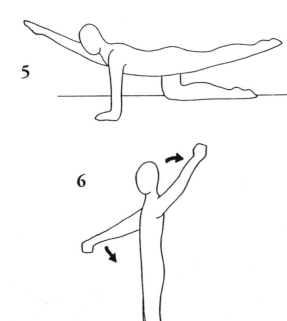

5. From a position on your hands and knees, raise your right arm and left leg as high as possible. Lower them and raise your left arm and right leg as high as possible and lower them. Continue in this way for 3 Minutes. Musically chant SA-TA-NA-MA in time with the movement and continue for another 3 Minutes. This movement can balance the lower back.

6. Stand up straight. Make your hands into fists. With the elbows straight, circle the arms in opposite directions. While one arm goes in a forward circle, the other arm goes in a backward circle. Rapidly chant "Har, Har, Har, Haree" in coordination with the movement. 2 Minutes. This movement can balance the rib cage. To finish, circle both arms in the same direction for about 15 seconds.

7. Sit down in Easy Pose and raise the arms up. Vigorously shake your arms, shoulders, and upper torso. Powerfully shake every part of you into adjustment. 1 Minute.

8. Still in Easy Pose, place your fists on the floor next to your hips. Bounce up and down on your buttocks. Chant "Har" each time your buttocks hit the floor. Chanting should be quick and continuous: "Har, Har, Har, Har." 30 seconds.

9. Lie down and relax. 11 Minutes.

This is a strenuous set of exercises. Exercise 2 is especially demanding. Start by practicing exercise 2 for 3 minutes and gradually work up to the full 11 minutes. Relax at least one minute between exercises.

"Yoga is a science of reality and experiential proof of the sacredness of all life". YB

6

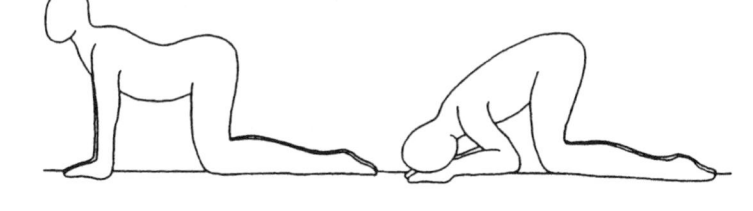

1

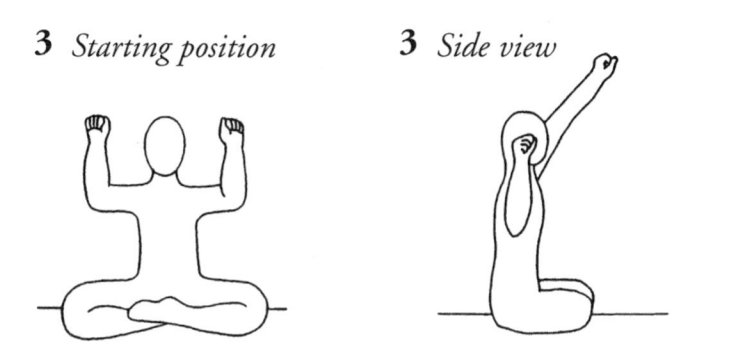

3 *Starting position*   **3** *Side view*

Center Line

3 *Top view*   *45°*

Creating Internal Balance

June 5, 1984

1. Sit in Easy Pose with your upper arms close to your sides. Your elbows are bent and your forearms extend forward, parallel to the floor. The palms are down. Begin moving your forearms up and down together, as if you are bouncing a ball. This movement is heavy, powerful, and rhythmic. The breath will automatically become a Breath of Fire in harmony with the strength of the movement. 4 Minutes.

2. Come on to your hands and knees in Cow Pose. Place your hands side by side on the floor so that they are centered under your chest. Bow down, touching your forehead to the backs of both hands. Rise back up into Cow Pose with your elbows straight. Continue this movement vigorously with a powerful breath. 4 Minutes. This exercise energizes the brain.

3. Sit in Easy Pose with your upper arms out to the sides and parallel to the floor. Your elbows are bent and your forearms extend upward. Make fists with your hands. Keeping the left arm in place, stretch the right arm up at a sixty degree angle and bring it back. Now keep the right arm in place as you stretch the left arm up at a sixty degree angle and bring it back. (Your arm should stretch diagonally forward as it goes up, so that, at its fullest extension, it forms a sixty degree angle to your body's center line as well as a sixty degree angle upward.) Make your fists heavy. Breathe heavily and move fast. The body will sway with the movement. The shoulders and ribcage will move. 3 1/2 Minutes.

4

5

4. Sit in Easy Pose with your elbows bent and your hands on your shoulders. The elbows are up and slightly forward. Alternately lean left and right. Sway the entire body to the same degree, do not bend your neck separately. Move powerfully. 2 Minutes.

5. Sit in Easy Pose with your fingers interlaced and your arms forming a hoop in front of your heart center. Your hands are about twelve inches from your chest. Find your own balance point. Move the navel without the breath. Inhale, vigorously pump your navel as long as you can. Then exhale, and vigorously pump your navel. Develop a pace and rhythm that will sustain you. 3 Minutes.

Close your eyes and concentrate at the brow point and continue pumping your navel. 4 Minutes.

Continue pumping your navel and begin to flex your spine like you are riding a horse. 2 1/2 Minutes.

For the next 1 1/2 Minutes chant "Har Har" with the tip of your tongue each time you pump your navel. Move the navel and chant as fast as you can. Try to chant "Har Har" eighty-four times during this time.

To finish: Inhale deeply, hold your breath for 30 seconds, and exhale. Repeat this sequence two more times.

Exercise can bring you emotional release and can tire you out so you can sleep. You exert yourself, sweat, and then deeply relax. This is very good, but, to achieve your total excellence, you must be able to control the chemistry of the blood. That is where Kundalini Yoga comes in. It is only through control of the chemistry of the blood, that one can sustain one's excellence over the long run. Glands are the guardians of your health and their secretions are vital to the strength and emotional balance needed in life.

"If the glandular secretion and the blood chemistry are not right, it doesn't matter how powerful and wonderful you are, you are a handicapped person."
YB

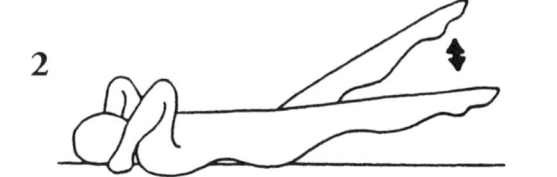

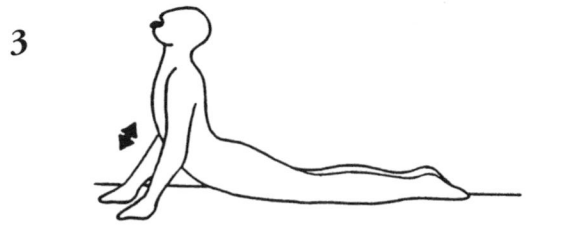

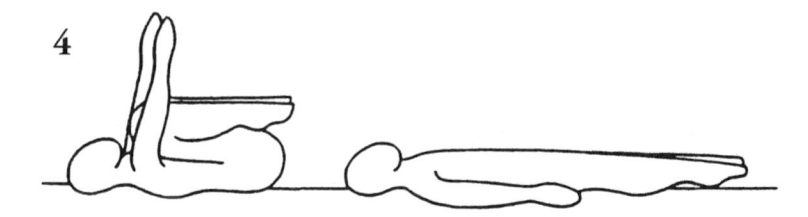

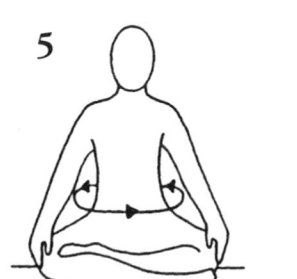

Detoxification

May 29, 1984

1. Lie down on your back with your legs straight. Your heels are together and your toes point upward. Keeping your heels together, spread your feet apart so that they both point out to the sides. The right foot points to the right and the left foot points to the left. Then close your feet so they once again point straight upward. Continue quickly opening and closing your feet, keeping your heels together. 4 Minutes.

2. Remain on your back and put your hands under your head. Raise your legs up about two feet and scissor the legs up and down without letting the descending heel touch the ground. Keep your legs straight, do not bend at the knees. This exercise clears up inner anger when done vigorously. 4 Minutes.

3. Lie down on your stomach and stick out your tongue. Exhale through your mouth and push up into Cobra Pose. Inhale through your mouth as you lower yourself back to the ground. Continue, keeping your breath and movement strong. This exercise removes toxins from the body. 6 1/2 Minutes.

4. Turn over on your back and bring your knees up to your chest. As the knees touch the chest, raise your arms up to 90 degrees (parallel to each other). Straighten your legs and lower your arms and legs back to the floor at the same time. Continue this movement vigorously. 3 Minutes. This is a controlled movement. There should be no noise when the arms and legs touch the ground.

5. Sit in Easy Pose and revolve the torso around the base of the spine. This churning movement is done in a counter-clockwise direction. Move as quickly as you can during the last minute. 3 Minutes.

"We detoxify continuously throughout life. We process food, thoughts, and all forms of energy. When that flow is continuous and clear, we are steady and flexible. The trouble is that we accumulate more than we process. We become weighted down under the ash of metabolism and the remnants of old emotions. This set systematically moves the energy of the body and mind to keep you light and vitalized." GCSK

6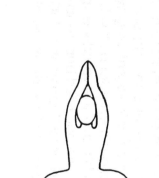

6. Stand up. Bend over and grab your ankles. While holding onto your ankles, sit down in Crow Pose and come back up. Continue this movement for 2 Minutes.

7. Sit comfortably in Easy Pose with your spine straight. Chant "Sat Nam, Sat Nam, Sat Nam, Sat Nam, Sat Nam, Sat Nam, Wahe Guru". (One full repetition of the mantra takes 7-8 seconds.) 11 Minutes.

To finish: Inhale deeply and stretch your arms over your head with your palms touching. Hold your breath 20-40 seconds as you stretch your spine upward. Exhale. Repeat this sequence two more times.

"A yogi is one whom the pair of opposites does not affect. He does not obey the law of duality and polarity." YB

7

To finish

Firing Up the Metabolism

March 6, 1985

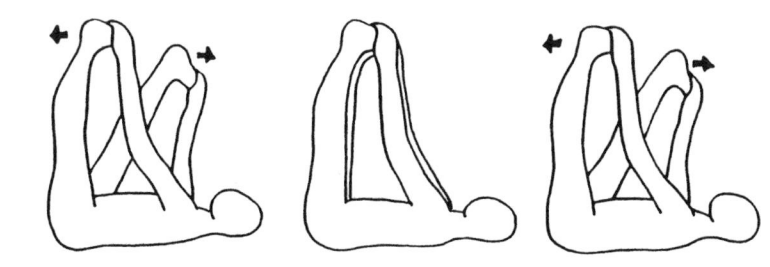

1. Lie down on your back. Raise your legs toward the ceiling and grasp your toes. Keep your legs up while you open and close them rapidly. Do Breath of Fire, timing the breath with the opening and closing of the legs. 5 1/2 Minutes.

2. Remain in the same position, holding onto your toes with your legs up. Pull your left leg toward your head. Let your left leg go back to the starting position as you pull your right leg toward your head. Continue alternately moving your legs up and down. Breath of Fire through the nose. 2 Minutes.

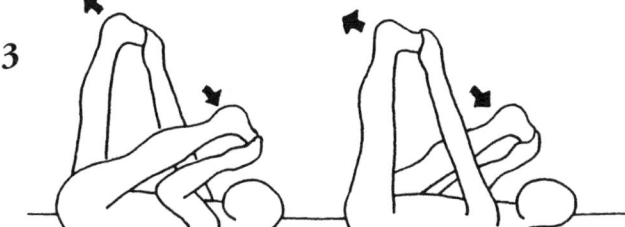
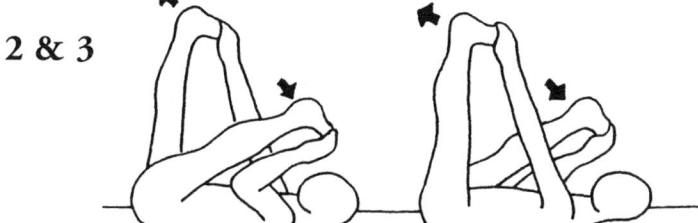

3. Continue the previous movement chanting "Har" with the tip of the tongue as each leg moves. Chant at a rate of two "Har's" per second. 12 Minutes.

4. Stay in the same position and combine the movements of exercises 1 and 2. Chant "Har" as your left leg moves up and down. Chant "Har" as your right leg moves up and down. Chant "Mukande" as you open and close your legs. One repetition of "Har, Har, Mukande" takes 2 seconds. Move quickly. 1 1/2 Minutes.

5. Sit up and relax for 1 Minute.

"There is a special fire within you that is the heat of the spirit. Its brilliance chases away all darkness and its clarity shows you the way to your soul".
GCSK

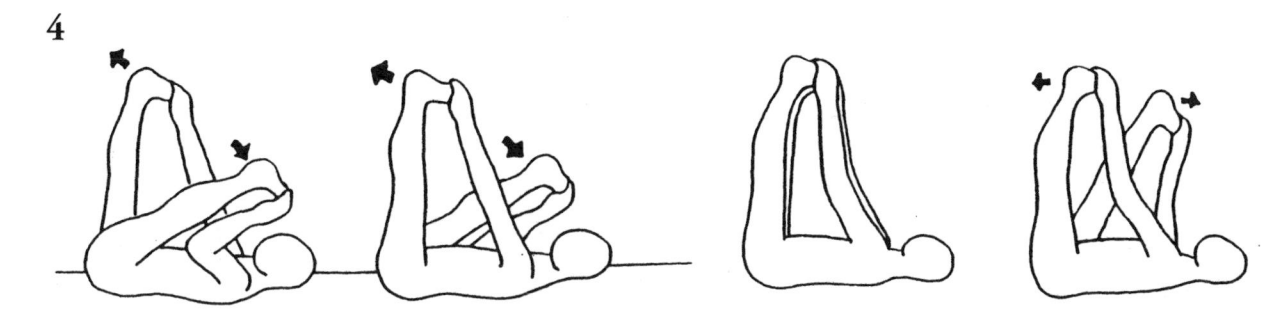

6

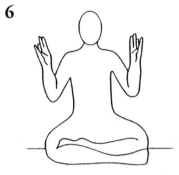

6. Sit in Easy Pose with the elbows bent and the palms facing forward at the level of the shoulders. The thumb and Sun finger touch in Surya Mudra. Close your eyes and chant "Har, Har, Mukande" rhythmically and musically for 11 Minutes. One repetition of the mantra takes 2 seconds.

To finish: Inhale and repeat this affirmation:

Let thy soul be awakened.

Let thy soul be awakened.

Let thy soul be awakened.

Let thy soul be awakened.

Let thy soul be awakened.

Let the Guru's lotus feet be in your heart.

Let the Guru's lotus feet be in your heart.

Let the Guru's lotus feet be in your heart.

Let the Guru's lotus feet be in your heart.

Let the lotus feet of the Guru be in your heart.

Let the lotus feet of the Guru be in your heart.

Let the lotus feet of the Guru be in your heart.

Let the lotus feet of the Guru be in your heart.

Let the lotus feet of the Guru be in your heart.

Wake up. Wake up. Wake up. Wake up. Wake up. Wake up. Wake up.

Heal. Heal. Heal. Heal.

Excel, excel, excel, excel, excel, excel, excel.

Obey, serve.

Obey, serve, love, excel. Obey, serve, love, excel

Obey, serve, love, excel Obey, serve, love, excel.

"Just see how powerful a mantra can be. All these stars and all this universe are very powerful, I am not dis-agreeing with the powers... but, by chanti-ng a mantra, just see how powerful you can be". YB

1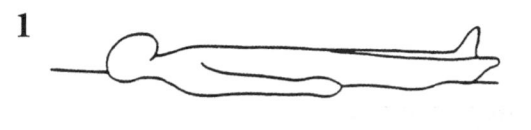

2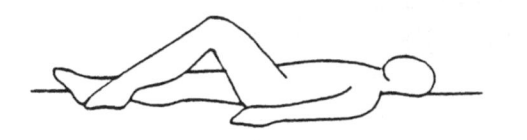

January 31, 1986

A Wake-up Set

3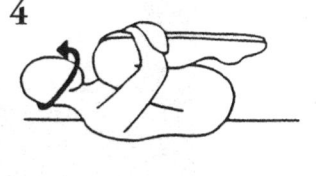

These exercises may be done on those mornings when you feel too tired to get up and go to work:

1. Lie on your back and move your feet alternately forward and back at the ankles, pointing and flexing the feet. 30 Seconds.

2. Raise and lower your knees alternately. 30 Seconds. Sometimes while sleeping, the circulation in the lower body becomes sluggish.

3. Still lying on your back, move your shoulders from side to side, sliding back and forth like a snake. 1 Minute.

4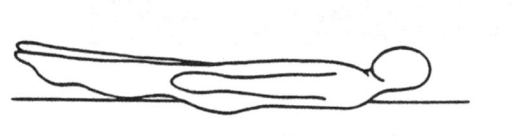

4. Clasp your knees to your chest with your arms. Lift your head and roll it around. 30 Seconds.

5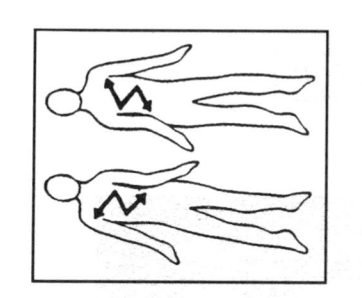

5. Raise your head and heels six inches, arms at your sides in Stretch Pose. Hold this position until your navel starts to jump and you don't want to stay up any longer. Relax. Repeat this exercise two more times. (You can do this exercise either three times total or for three minutes, whichever is shorter.)

6. Lie on your back and stretch left and right in Cat Stretch. 30 Seconds.

6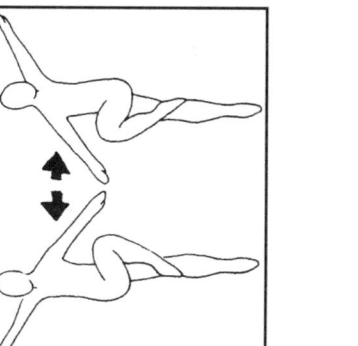

7. Sit up with your legs stretched out straight. Grab your toes. Raise and lower your torso, bringing your head to your knees. 30 Seconds.

7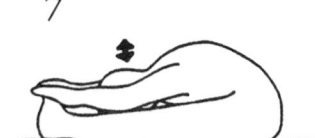

Recharge Yourself

 1

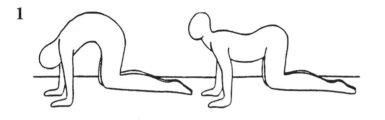

1. On your hands and knees, do Cat-Cow with breath of fire. 1 1/2 Minutes.

2. Sit in easy pose and reach your left arm straight out in front. Then reach your right arm straight out in front as you twist your torso to the left pulling your left arm in. Continue. Twist your torso and shoulders left and right as if you are pulling a heavy rope. Move vigorously. 3 Minutes.

"Don't become spiritual for my sake. I didn't become spiritual for anybody's sake. I became spiritual for my own sake". YB

3. Rock back and forth on your stomach in Bow Pose with Breath of Fire. 3 Minutes.

4. Stand up with your arms straight out in front, palms facing down. Sit down and stand up again. 20 Times.

5. Sit in easy pose with your arms stretched up over your head, palms together. Chant your favorite mantra. 2 Minutes. Inhale and stretch up. Exhale and relax.

6. Lie down on your stomach and sleep. 11-21 Minutes.

2

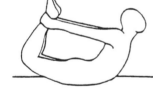

3

4

5

14

Overcoming Weakness

January 9, 1985

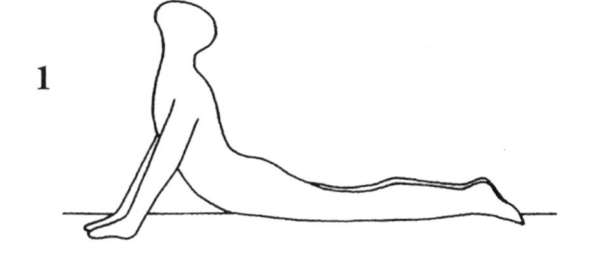

1. Come into Cobra Pose, heels together, elbows straight and chin tilted upward. 3 1/2 Minutes. Remain in the same posture, put your tongue out and begin a powerful, panting breath from the diaphragm. 2 Minutes. Still in cobra pose, pull in your tongue, close your mouth, and begin Breath of Fire through your nose. 2 Minutes.

Slowly come out of the posture.

2. Lie down and relax on your stomach. 1 Minute.

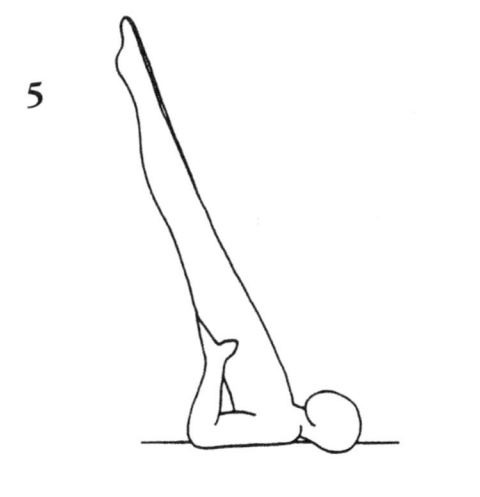

3. Grab your ankles and stretch up into Bow Pose. Inhale through your mouth and exhale through your nose. 5 Minutes. (The muscles in your thighs and pelvis regulate the mineral balance in the body, so pain in your thighs during this exercise can indicate a calcium/magnesium imbalance.)

4. Relax on your back. 6 Minutes.

5. Come up into a variation of Shoulder Stand. Using your hands to support your lower back firmly, angle your torso up to sixty degrees. Extend your legs up and out so that they are in a straight line with your torso and there is no bend in your back. Keep your knees straight. The forward angle of your torso and legs puts the weight of your body on to your elbows. Stick your tongue out and do Breath of Fire through your mouth. 3 Minutes.

6. Come into Stretch Pose. Lift your head and heels 6 inches and extend your arms over your thighs, palms down. Focus your eyes at the tips of your toes. Do Breath of Fire and really pump your navel point. 2 1/2 Minutes. (Three minutes a day of Stretch Pose is very good for your liver.)

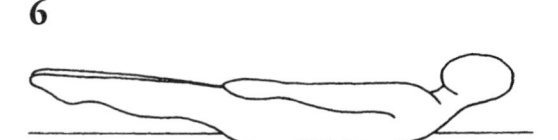

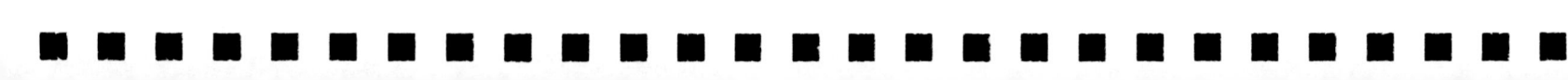

7. Relax on your back. 6 Minutes.

8. Roll your hands and feet. Move your elbows, shoulders, and shoulder blades. Gradually begin to move more and more until you are moving around wildly, shaking energy into every cell. Experience your power over your own weakness, laziness and sluggishness. 1 1/2 Minutes.

"God is within you. It was. It is. It shall be".
YB

DRINK FOR BALANCING THE MINERALS IN YOUR BODY:

Soak 6 prunes, 6 figs, and a handful of raisins in water overnight. In the morning add 3 bananas and 8 ounces of yoghurt. Blend altogether in a blender with some ice and the water in which you soaked the fruit. Divide this mixture into three equal portions and drink throughout the day. (If you wish to make this drink a complete food, add a handful of nuts before blending. Those who suffer from cold hands and cold feet may add 10-15 soaked saffron threads as well.) You may want to drink this drink daily instead of eating your regular meals. If so, every other day, you must eat a large meal of steamed vegetables or a hearty vegetable salad in addition to the drinks.

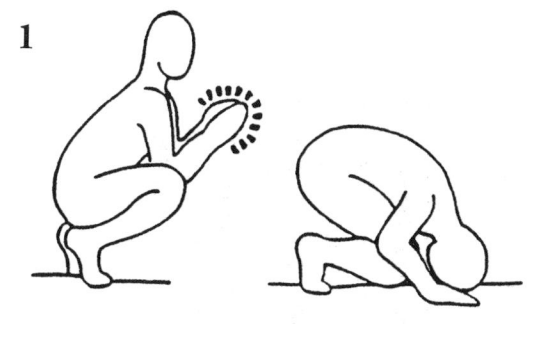

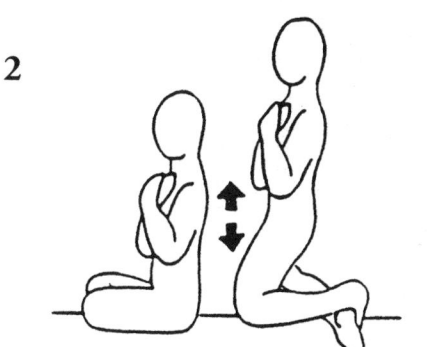

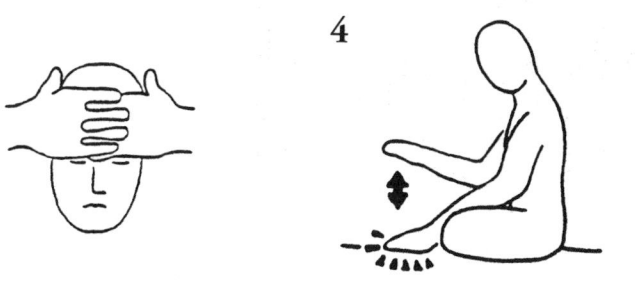

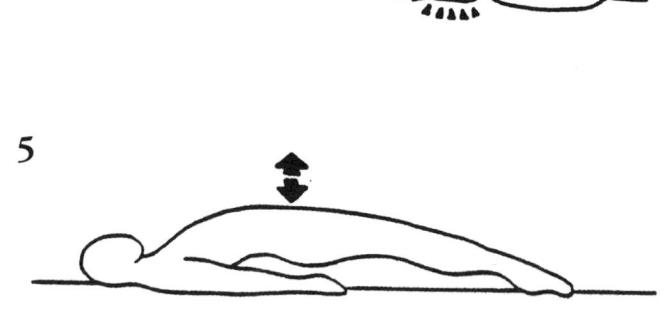

Preparing Yourself Physically, Mentally, and Spiritually

March 5, 1986

1. Sit on your heels with your knees spread wide, balancing on the balls of your feet as in Frog Pose. Clap your hands once and then bend from the waist, touching your forehead to the floor. Return to the starting position and continue clapping and bowing. 2 Minutes.

2. Sit in Easy Pose and cross your hands over your heart. Your left hand is against your chest and your right hand is on top of your left hand. Keeping your legs crossed as in Easy Pose and your hands on your heart, raise yourself up so that you are balanced on your knees and then drop back down into Easy Pose. Move rapidly up and down. This modified body drop is good for your heart. 6 Minutes.

3. Lie down on your back. Interlock your fingers and hold your forehead. The base of the palms press against your temples and your thumbs are pointing upward toward the top of your head. Keep your hands in this position as you twist and turn and move every part of your body. Imagine that you are in great pain and move vigorously. 1 1/2 Minutes.

4. Sit in Easy Pose. Look at the ground in front of you as you beat the ground with your open palms. Keep your hands open. Move hard and fast, work out any stored anger. 1 1/2 Minutes.

5. Lie down on your back. Quickly raise and lower your buttocks, creating an invigorating massage. Move quickly. This exercise is to open up the pelvic area. It stimulates the juncture of the two sciatic nerves of the legs. This stimulation is needed for the pituitary to function properly. 2 Minutes.

6. Remain on your back and immediately put yourself into a deep, relaxing nap. 4 Minutes. Gradually rise up and sing along with "Dhan, Dhan Ram Das Gur" on *Naad the Blessing* by Sangeet Kaur. 7 Minutes.

"It is a daily requirement that the body's energies be properly stimulated so you can live smoothly, think smoothly, and go through the day gracefully and peacefully". YB

Recuperate the Inner Organs

October 10, 1984

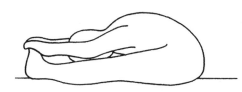

1. Make your hands into fists and place them on your shoulders close to your neck. Raise your elbows as high as you can. Focus at the tip of your nose. Breathe deeply and powerfully through your nose, making sure to expand your upper lungs. Fill your lungs to their capacity. 5 Minutes.

If the lungs are not filled with oxygen, then the oxygen supply in the blood is minimal and natural depression becomes part of you.

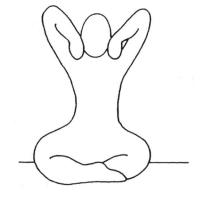

2. Lie down flat on your back. Put your heels together and stretch your toes forward. Make a "V" of your body by raising both your legs and torso up to approximately sixty degrees. Your arms are stretched out in front of you at whatever angle allows you to stay balanced. The palms are down and the elbows are straight. The exact position will vary from person to person. Breathe strongly and deeply. Hold this position for 8 Minutes.

The navel point will vibrate heavily and adjust the energy throughout the glandular system.

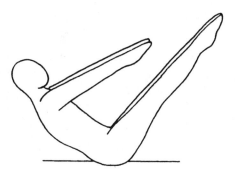

3. Stretch your legs out in front of you, grab your toes, bend your torso forward, bringing your head down to your knees and rise back up. Chant "Har, Har, Har, Har, Har, Har, Haree" in coordination with this up and down movement. 2 1/2 Minutes.

4. Lie down on your back and relax. Let your life concentrate at your navel point. 10 Minutes.

5. Still lying down, chant "Har, Har, Har, Har, Har, Har, Har, Har, Har, Har, Har, Har, Wahe Guru". 1 Minute.

6. Cat Stretch left and right. Stretch every part of your body.

"A Teacher brings God into the heart of another person". YB

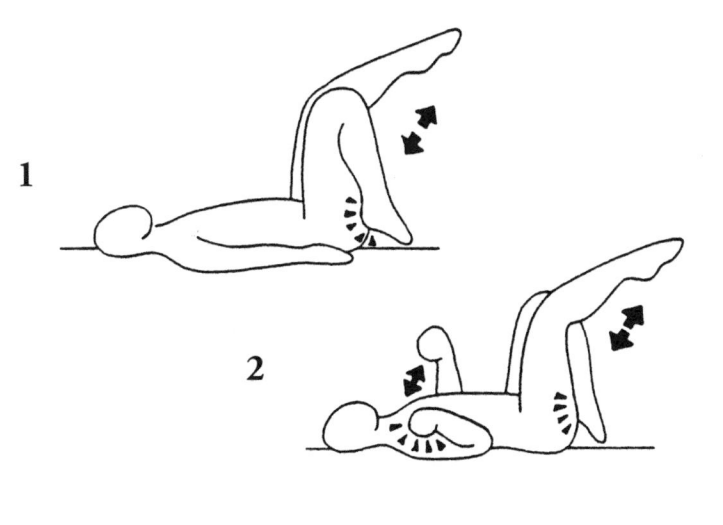

To Release Stored Pain and Refresh Yourself

February 27, 1985

1. Lie down flat on your back. Bend your knees and begin kicking your buttocks. Kick alternately with your left and right heels. 5 1/2 Minutes. During the last minute move as fast as you can. Move directly into exercise 2.

2. Continue alternately kicking your buttocks. Bend your arms at the elbows and alternately hit your shoulders with your fists, rhythmically coordinating the movements of arms and legs. Your hands do not hit the ground. 2 Minutes. Move fast.

3. Still lying on your back, Cat Stretch left and right, quickly alternating from side to side. 2 1/2 Minutes.

4. Sit up in Easy Pose and put your hands lightly on the top of your head. Twist your torso left and right, moving with force and speed. 2 Minutes.

5. Put your hands on your knees and rotate your head in a figure eight. Move quickly and powerfully. 30 Seconds.

6. Lie down on your back and relax. Concentrate on your pituitary gland at the brow point. Breathe through your nose slowly and deeply. 7 1/2 Minutes. Next move your concentration to your navel point. Mentally chant along with *Jaap Sahib, Last Four Lines,* by Kulwant Singh, pulling your navel point in with the beat. 9 Minutes.

This last part can be done by itself as a meditation. Lie down on your back and pull your navel in with the rhythm of this tape of *Jaap Sahib, Last Four Lines* . "One tape can do a miracle. Seven days a week can do it for your life."

Chattar Chakkar Vartee, Chattar Chakkar Bhugatay

Suyambhav Subhang, Sarab Daa Sarab Jugatay

Dukaalang Pranaasee, Dayaalang Saroopay

Sadaa Ang Sangay, Abhangang Bibhootay

"Either you have to please the moment or the Master. If you please the moment at the expense of the Master, you are a failure. If you please the Master, you are a success." YB

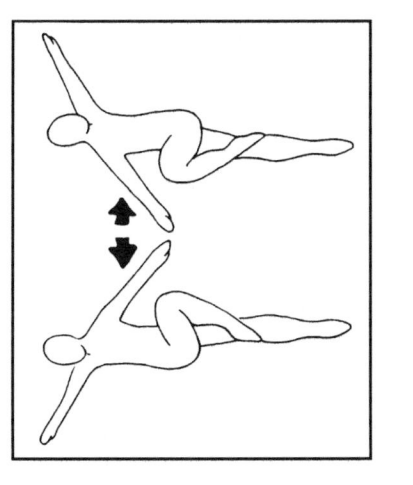

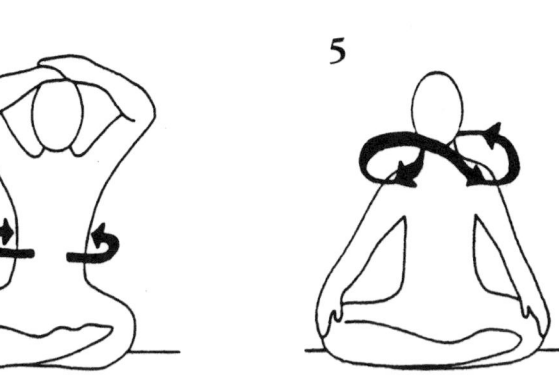

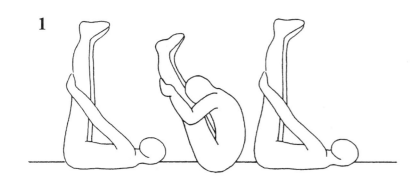

1

Take Charge of the Energy of Life

October 3, 1984

1. Lie down on your back. Raise both legs up to ninety degrees. Lock your hands together a little above the backs of your knees. Inhale, raise your upper body and touch your nose to your knees while holding your breath to your capacity. Exhale and lie back down keeping your legs up at ninety degrees. Continue raising and lowering your upper body in this way for 3 Minutes.

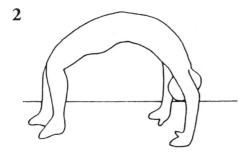

2

2. Lie on your back. Put your hands under your shoulders with the palms on the ground. Bend your knees and, keeping the soles of your feet on the floor, bring your heels near your buttocks. Carefully raise your pelvis until you are in Half Wheel Pose. Do Breath of Fire. 3 Minutes. This exercise puts pressure on the lymph glands. It is the only way you can work them out.

3. Come into Shoulder Stand. Inhale and lower your left foot to the floor behind your head. Keep your knees straight. Exhale and lower your right foot to the floor as you raise your left leg back up. Continue for 2 Minutes with long, deep breathing. Then begin Breath of Fire and move as fast as you can for the last 1 Minute.

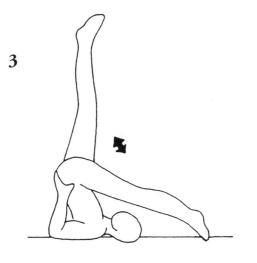

3

4. Return to a sitting posture. Close your eyes and meditate for 15 Minutes with long, deep breathing. Give strength to your pituitary and it will give you a wonderful day.

Examine how differently you feel after doing these exercises for just 3 minutes each. If you do exercise 1 for thirty-one times minimum, holding your breath to your capacity, it will make you a new person.

"You can either be above the energy of your life and ride it or you can be below the energy and it rides you. This is where Kundalini yoga fits in. It teaches you how to ride the energy."
YB

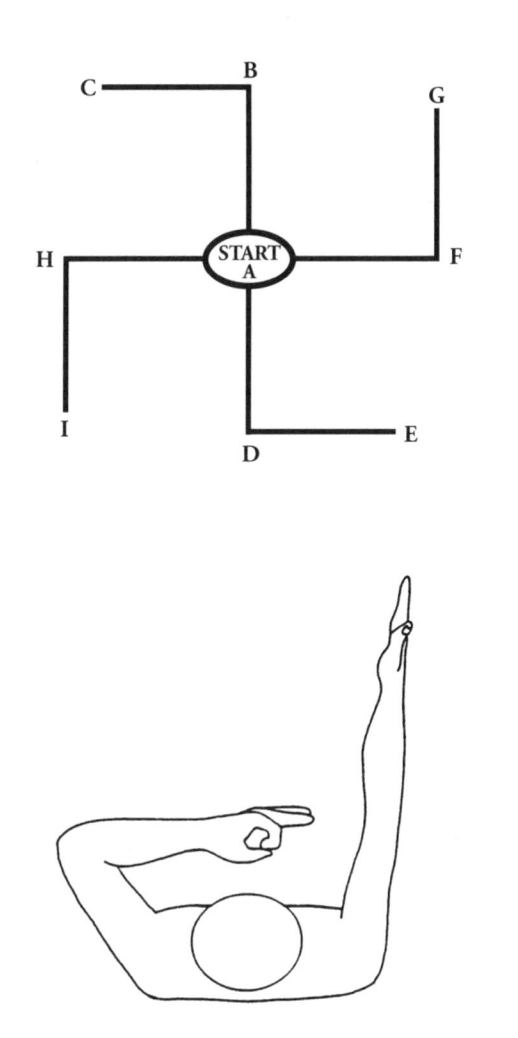

Right Hand

The Sun Wheel Meditation
A Salutation to God for the Purification of the Psyche

January 8, 1986

Swastika is a Sanskrit word meaning "well-being" or "good fortune". The symbol itself is also known as the Sun Wheel, and has been used as a mystical symbol since pre-historic times. The positive form of this symbol revolves in a counter-clockwise manner and means "toward God". The negative form revolves in a clockwise manner and means "away from God". The negative form was adopted by the Nazis, and, to the Western mind, both forms have come to symbolize evil and ill-will. This is unfortunate because, as you will experience in the following meditation, the positive form of this symbol has great power to uplift and purify.

1. Sit in Easy Pose and put your left hand in Gyan Mudra, keeping the Saturn, Sun, and Mercury fingers straight. Your left palm faces the chest at the heart center. Your left forearm is parallel to the floor. Your right arm is extended at shoulder level with the palm facing to the left and the thumb pointing upward. There is no bend in the right elbow during the movements. Sit straight, with your chin in and chest out.

Arm Movement: Pretend that the diagram illustration is painted on the wall in front of you and then use your arm to trace the pattern of the diagram in the air. You will be using your right arm to draw a counter-clockwise Sun Wheel in the air in front of your body.

To do this you will move your right arm in specific horizontal and vertical movements. Each movement is approximately 8". When the movement is <u>horizontal,</u> the palm of the hand faces <u>downward.</u> When the movement is <u>vertical,</u> the palm of the hand faces to the <u>left.</u>

■ ■

Moving your right arm: From the starting position A, turn your palm to the left, and move your arm vertically 8" to B. Turn your palm down and move horizontally 8" to the left to C. Move your arm horizontally back to the right to B. Turn your palm to the left and move vertically back to the starting point A.

From A, move your arm down vertically 8" to D. Turn your palm down and move horizontally 8" to the right to E. Move your arm back horizontally to the left to D. Turn the palm to the left and move vertically back up to A.

From A, turn your palm down and move horizontally 8" to the right to F. Turn your palm to the left and move vertically 8" up to G. Move vertically back down to F. Turn your palm down and move horizontally back to the starting position A.

From A, move horizontally to the left 8" to H. Turn your palm to the left and move vertically down 8" to I. Move vertically back up to H. Turn your palm down and move horizontally back to the starting position A.

Continue this sequence, breathing slowly and deeply. Begin with 3 minutes using the right arm to make the Sun Wheel and then do the same movement using the left arm for 3 minutes. Gradually work up to 31 minutes on each side. It is permissible to do one side of the meditation in the morning and the other side in the evening.

When you change to the left arm, it is very important that the Sun Wheel is still in the same pattern you made with the right arm. In other words, the symbol still revolves counter-clockwise. The arm changes but the pattern of the Sun Wheel remains the same as the diagram.

When you change to the left arm, the palm will face to the _right_ when the movement is _vertical_.

"The beauty of Kundalini Yoga is that it is a technique to move the psyche through a physical force." YB

22

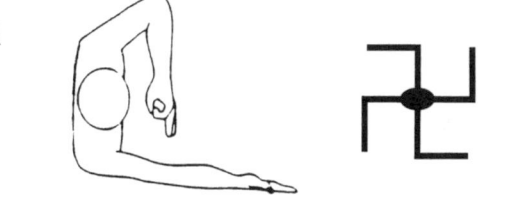

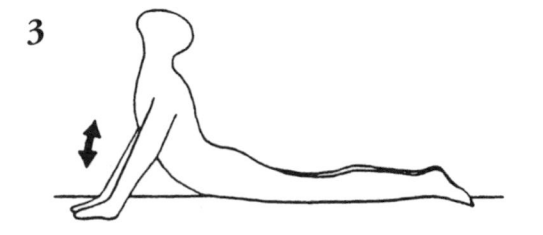

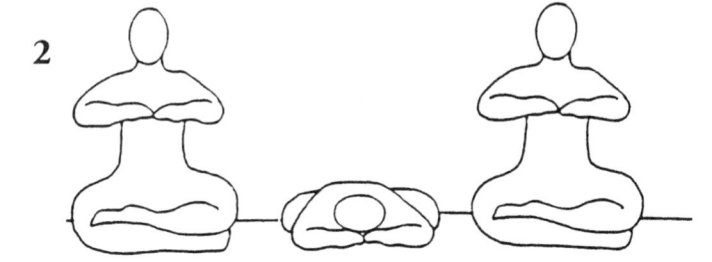

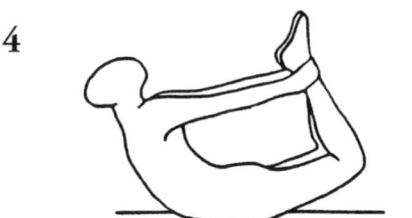

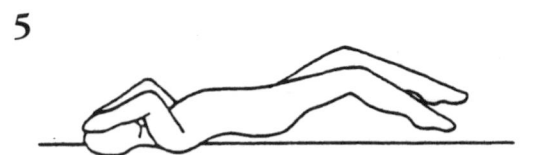

Heal Your Troubles

January 8, 1986

To practice this kriya, you will need a banana.

1. Sun Wheel Meditation. 1-3 Minutes on each side.

2. Sit in Easy Pose. Your elbows are bent and your forearms are parallel to the floor. Your palms face downward with the tips of the fingers of one hand touching the tips of the fingers of the other hand. (Which fingertips actually touch will depend on the length of your fingers.) Maintain this arm position and bend forward until your hands touch the floor and your forehead touches the backs of your hands. Rise back up into the starting position, sitting straight.

This movement is combined with the breath. For each breath cycle: inhale deeply, hold the breath, bow and rise up a total of 16 times, and then exhale to complete one breath cycle. Move quickly but rise up completely after each bow. Do a total of 15 complete breath cycles.

3. Come into Cobra Pose. Inhale, hold your breath, bring your forehead to the ground and arch back up into Cobra Pose 16 times with your breath held. Then exhale to complete one breath cycle. Move fast, but make sure that you arch back up fully into Cobra Pose each time. Do 4 complete breath cycles.

4. Reach back, grab your ankles, and arch up into Bow Pose. Inhale, hold your breath, and roll forward and back on your stomach 16 times. Exhale to complete one breath cycle. Do 3 complete breath cycles.

5. Lie on your back with your hands on your forehead. Vigorously bounce and shake every part of your body. 1 Minute.

"To end your troubles, first establish a new pattern-one of balance and sacredness. Then speed up your elimination and clear away all fears and blocks. Finally, bless yourself and accept the blessing of the One in All." GCSK

7

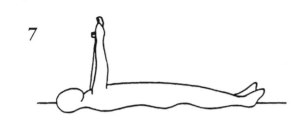

8

9

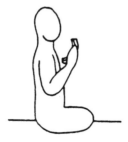

6. Lie on your back and breathe slowly and deeply from your navel. 7 Minutes. (During this meditation, Yogi Bhajan played the gong as the class listened to Bhai Avtar Singh and Bhai Gurucharan Singh's *Jai Te Gung* for 4 minutes followed by Singh Kaur's *Wahe Guru Jio* for 3 minutes.)

7. Still lying on your back, hold your banana lengthwise between your palms and raise your arms straight up in the air. Breathe slowly and deeply. Keep your arms straight and imagine that you are sanctifying and purifying the banana, filling it with healing energy. 3 Minutes.

8. Rise up into a sitting position with your arms stretched up straight over your head. The banana is still held vertically between your palms. Hold this position for a few seconds and then bend forward, stretching your hands toward your toes. Make a prayer as if you are offering something to God. This whole sequence takes about 30 seconds.

9. Sit in Easy Pose. Bring your hands to your chest in Prayer Mudra at your heart center with the banana still held vertically between your palms and pray. 10 Seconds.

10. Eat your banana. If you make this set of exercises a regular part of your life, eating the banana as your breakfast, you will have a lot less trouble in your life. The banana will act to balance the minerals and other elements in your body. It is a very essential food of life.

"To learn this kriya, I had to go to an ashram for six months and work. I brought forty to fifty 18# canisters of water every three hours. You understand how painful it is to learn from these old-time Masters?" YB

Work on the Hypothalamus

April 10; 1985

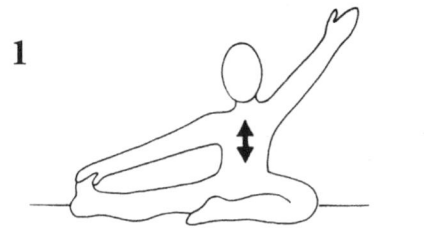

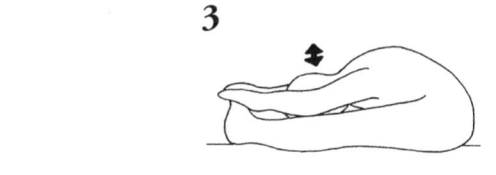

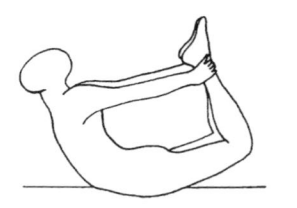

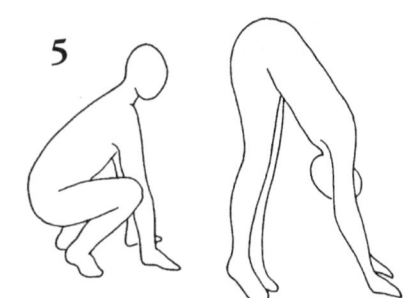

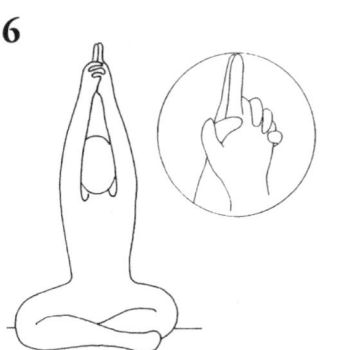

1. Sit in Easy Pose. Stretch your left arm diagonally out from your body. It is not straight out to the side nor straight out in front but in between these two positions. Raise the arm up to sixty degrees. Stretch your right leg out straight and grab the toes with your right hand. From this position lower your forehead to the floor and back up 108 times.

2. Reverse sides and repeat the first exercise 108 times.

3. Stretch both legs out in front of you and grab your toes with your hands. Raise and lower your torso bringing your forehead to your knees 108 times.

4. Lie down on your stomach in Bow Pose and rock back and forth 108 times.

5. Frog Pose. 108 times.

6. Sit in Easy Pose. Stretch your arms up over your head with the hands locked together. Concentrate at your brow point. Keep your elbows straight and your spine stretched.
Chant along with the tape *Har Har Mukande* by Avtar Singh.
Chant "Har, Har" from the navel and chant "Mukande" with the tip of your tongue. 7 1/2 Minutes.

To finish: Inhale deeply, hold your breath 25 seconds and stretch all twenty-six vertebra upward. Exhale. Repeat this sequence two more times.

7. Lie down and completely relax 11 Minutes.

"Life is a flow of love." YB

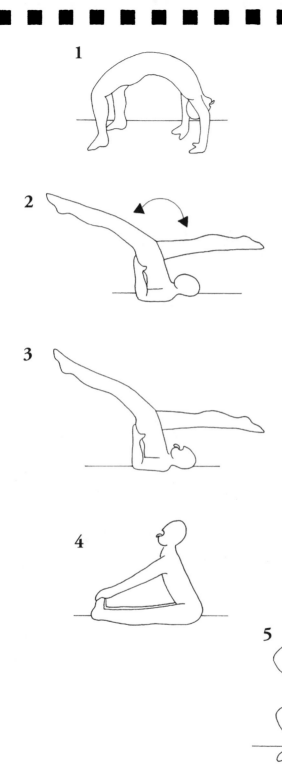

You and Your Body

February 13, 1985

1. Carefully come into Half Wheel Pose. Extend your tongue all the way out and do Breath of Fire through your mouth. 4 1/2 Minutes. Then slowly come out of the posture. Half Wheel Pose will show you exactly what kind of relationship exists between you and your body.

2. Come into Shoulder Stand with your hands supporting your hips. Bring your left leg back toward the floor behind you as you bring your right leg forward toward the floor in front. Continue alternately moving the legs in this way. 1 1/2 Minutes.

3. Freeze the motion of exercise 2 with your right leg backward and your left leg forward. 1 Minute.

Extend your tongue out and do breath of fire through your mouth. 2 Minutes. This exercise affects the liver to get the anger out.

4. Sit with your legs stretched out straight in front of you. Grab your toes and straighten your spine. Lift your chin up toward the ceiling, extend your tongue and do Breath of Fire through your mouth. 1 1/2 Minutes.

5. Sit in Crow Pose and interlock your fingers on the top of your head. Chant quickly in a monotone using the tip of your tongue: "Hari Har, Hari Har, Hari Har Haree." 3 Minutes. (One round of the mantra will take about 3 seconds.)

6. Relax.

"The body is not your friend, not your enemy, not your identity. Body has no relationship with you. It is a time-wise momentary vehicle which gives you the right to live and experience life." YB

December 5, 1995

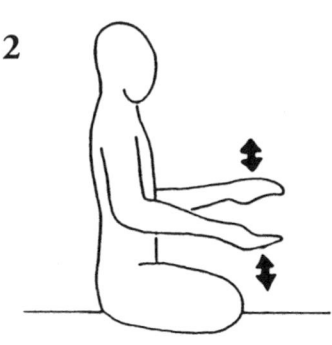

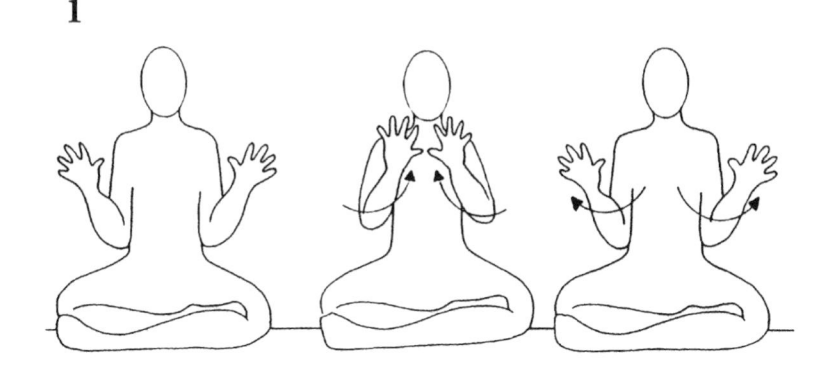

1. Sit in Easy Pose with your elbows bent, upper arms resting alongside the rib cage, and forearms pointing upward. Your palms face forward with the fingers spread. The fingers are straight and slightly stiff. Keep your palms facing forward as each hand moves in a small, U-shaped arc toward the center of the body and back out to the starting position at the sides. The thumbs do not touch in the center. Move fast. Close your eyes. Move at the speed of three in-and-out movements per second. The whole spine will move vigorously if you are doing the movement correctly. 6 Minutes.

To finish: inhale, hold your breath 10-15 seconds while you make fists of your hands and squeeze your entire body. Exhale. Repeat this sequence two more times.

This exercise will equalize the Tattwas in the body. Your circulation will be stimulated and the serum in your spine will rise.

2. Sit in Easy Pose with your elbows bent, upper arms alongside the rib cage, and forearms parallel to the ground. The right palm faces upward to the heavens and the left palm faces downward to the earth. The hands are slightly stiff. Move your forearms alternately a few inches up and down. When the left arm moves upward, the right arm moves downward and so on. This movement must be so powerful that your whole body shakes. The central core of your body must move about one inch with the power of the movement of your arms. Move vigorously. 4 1/2 Minutes.

To finish: Inhale, hold the breath 10 seconds, while you lock your back molars and squeeze your jaws. Exhale. Repeat this sequence two more times.

This exercise may be painful for those who have a tendency toward arthritis, but it can help alleviate that condition. It also aids digestion. You will develop a special breath for the last 15 seconds of the exercise if you are doing it correctly.

"Body is not all. Mind is not all. Spirit is not all. All three make the sense". YB

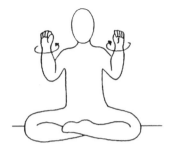

3 *Front View*

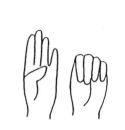

Mudra for 3

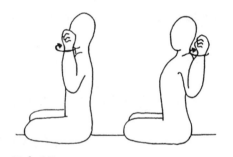

3 *Side View*

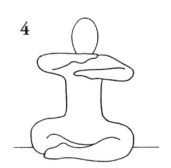

4

3. Sit in Easy Pose with your elbows bent, upper arms along rib cage and the forearms pointing upward. Place your thumbs on the mound of the Sun finger and make fists of your hands. Your fists face forward. Moving from the elbow, revolve your lower arms and hands in small inward circles toward the center of your chest. As you revolve your fists pull your shoulders back so that your shoulder blades come together and your chest is opened up. Then, while still making the circles, relax your shoulders forward. Alternate pulling the shoulders back for maximum stretch and relaxing them forward as you continue to make rapid inward circles with your fists. Close your eyes and move fast. 1 1/2 Minutes.

This adjusts the ribs and gives more oxygen to the blood. Inhale deeply and move gracefully into the next exercise.

4. Sit with your elbows bent and the forearms about shoulder height. The palms face downward. The right palm is over the left at the center of the body with about 4 inches of space between the hands. Close your eyes, breathe slowly and deeply, becoming calm and thoughtless. Give a rest to your intellect. Listen to the tape of *"Sat Nam Wahe Guru #2"* by Jagjit Singh and meditate on your essence. After 3 Minutes, begin chanting in a whisper along with the tape. Use the tip of the tongue along the upper palate, hissing the "S" sound with the force of the breath. Whisper the chant for 6 more minutes.

To finish: Inhale through your mouth slowly and deeply with a hiss and exhale through your mouth slowly and deeply with a hiss. Repeat this breath two more times.

As a regular practice, do each of these exercise for 3 minutes early every morning, instead of sleeping.

28

Ardas Bhaee

1-29-86

ARDAS BHAEE, AMAR DAS GURU
AMAR DAS GURU, ARDAS BHAEE
RAM DAS GURU
RAM DAS GURU
RAM DAS GURU
SACHEE SAHEE

"Normally there is no power in the human but the power of prayer. And to do prayer, you have to put your mind and body together and then pray from the soul. Ardas Bhaee is a mantra prayer. If you sing it, your mind, body and soul automatically combine and without saying what you want, the need of the life is adjusted. That is the beauty of this prayer."

Yogi Bhajan

Breath of Ten
Meditation to Become Disease-Free

May 8, 1995

Sit in Easy Pose with a straight spine. Your elbows are bent and your forearms and hands are relaxed and in a clapping position. Your hands move in and out like you are clapping but they do not touch. Stop the inward motion when the hands are about six to eight inches apart. Move slowly and rhythmically. Concentrate on the energy that you can feel between the palms of your hands.

The breath is timed with the movement of the hands. Inhale in five strokes through the nose and exhale in five strokes through the mouth. Each stroke of the breath is one clapping motion. Do not break the rhythm of the movement and breath. 16 1/2 Minutes.

To finish: Inhale deeply, hold your breath for 20 seconds as you press your hands against your face as hard as you can. Exhale. Inhale deeply, hold your breath for 20 seconds as you strongly press your hands against your heart center. Exhale. Inhale deeply, hold your breath for 20 seconds as you press your hands hard against your navel point. Exhale and relax.

This is magnetic energy therapy. The energy connection between the hands must not be broken. This exercise triggers the command center to wake up the immune system.

Do this meditation every day for 11 minutes and it will put all the chakras in rhythm.

"The Breath of Ten is a complete breath in the line of Breath of Fire. It can give you a disease-free body, a clear, meditative mind and develop your intuition, but it requires practice." YB

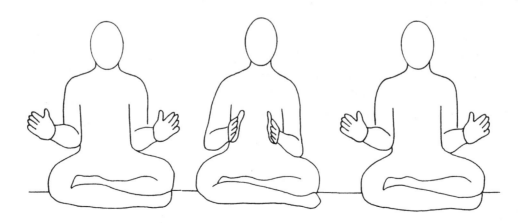

30

May 10, 1996

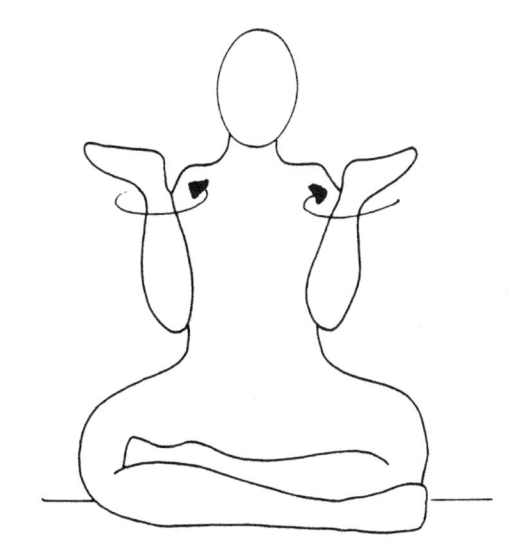

Top View

1. Sit in Easy Pose with your elbows bent so that your upper arms are alongside your rib cage and your elbows rest against the lower ribs. Your forearms point upward. The palms are flat and face the heavens. The fingers are firm. Move your forearms in small inward circles keeping the palms flat and facing upwards. Move from the elbow but keep the elbows resting on the lower ribs. As you move your eyes will close automatically. Chant along with the tape of *Jaap Sahib-Last Four LInes* by Kulwant Singh.

Chattar Chakkar Vartee, Chattar Chakkar Bhugatay

Suyambhav Subhang, Sarab Daa Sarab Jugatay

Dukaalang Pranaasee, Dayaalang Saroopay

Sadaa Ang Sangay, Abhangang Bibhootay

Chant using the tip of your tongue against your upper palate. This will affect your thalamus and hypothalamus. 11-18 Minutes. "Once the thalamus and hypothalamus shall move, you shall have a different world to live in. You will enter a different horizon."

To finish: Inhale, hold your breath for 10-15 seconds, while making your inward circles as fast as you can (3 times per second) and exhale. Repeat this sequence two more times.

"This is the most sacred and secret kriya in all yoga. Out of it was born Buddhism, Hinduism, Kabballah, and all mysticism." YB

■ ■

Cleanse The Bloodstream

November 9, 1995

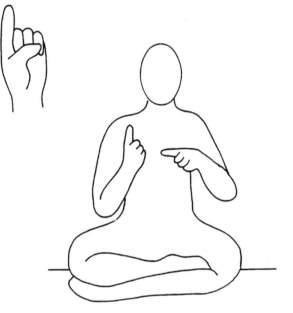

1. Sit in Easy Pose with your spine straight. Bend your elbows so that both hands are in front of your body near the heart center. Keep the Jupiter fingers pointing straight while using your thumbs to lock down the other fingers. The Jupiter finger of your right hand points straight up. The Jupiter finger of your left hand is parallel to the floor and points at the right thumb. Allow a space of six inches between the left Jupiter finger and the thumb of the right hand. (This space allows the flow of an electro-magnetic filament of energy.) Keep your chin in and your chest out. Close your eyes 9/10ths. Make a circle of your mouth. Deeply inhale through the O-shaped mouth. Exhale through your nose. 7 Minutes. This is a Jupiter meditation which can cleanse the bloodstream and relieve fatigue and tension if you breathe deeply and powerfully. It is this conscious breath that can bring you great relief.

"Live like a God. Give like an angel. Be a bright, beautiful, bountiful human being." YB

2. Stay in the same position and chant along with the tape of *Wahe Guru Jio* by Gyaniji. Chant using the tip of your tongue against your upper palate. 4 1/2 Minutes.

3. Begin to whisper the chant, concentrating on the mantra. After 30 seconds, Yogi Bhajan played Nirinjan Kaur's tape of "Every Heartbeat" while instructing the students to concentrate on their whispered chanting of the Wahe Jio mantra for an additional 3 Minutes.

4. Chant the mantra "Aad sach, Jugaad sach, Haibhay Sach, Nanak Hosee Bhay Sach". Concentrating on this mantra while continuing to listen to "Every Heartbeat." 1 1/2 Minutes.

To finish: Inhale, hold your breath 15-25 seconds, while stretching your spine upward. (This meditation relaxes you in such a way that you should be able to achieve more stretch in your spine than is usually possible. Really stretch the spine, concentrating on each vertebra.) Exhale and repeat this sequence two more times.

Conquer Pain

February 8, 1995

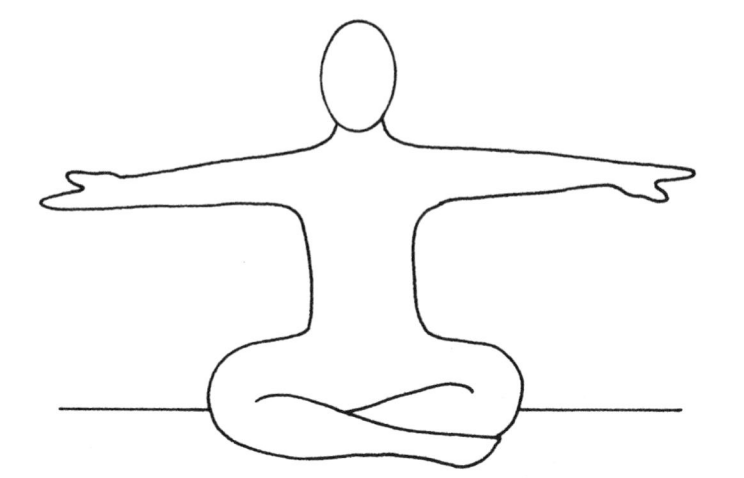

Sit in Easy Pose with your spine straight and your chin in and chest out. Split your fingers so that the Jupiter and Saturn fingers are together and the Sun and Mercury fingers are together. Stretch your arms straight out to the sides, parallel to the ground. There will be a stretch felt in the armpits. The left palm faces downward and the right palm faces upward. Inhale deeply and powerfully through the mouth as if you are drinking the air. Exhale powerfully through the nose. Slow your breathing so that you breathe only three times per minute. Keep your arms straight and your armpits stretched. 11 Minutes.

To finish: Inhale deeply through your mouth, hold your breath for 15 seconds, stretch your arms out to the sides, and stretch your spine upward. Exhale through the nose and repeat this sequence two more times.

This self-healing process builds your body's capacity to conquer pain. It balances your central nervous system.

After three minutes the pain will grow and you must be strong to conquer any negativity. There will be a war between you and your mind and you have to win it.

This kriya trains your body to fight pain. When your body is trained to fight pain, you can conquer any obstacle.

"Self doesn't rest. Self seeks."
YB

Experiencing The Psyche

December 15, 1993

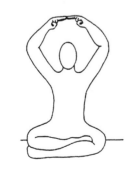

Before you begin this meditation, move your body all around to loosen up. You must be relaxed so you will not block the flow of energy. Feel good and comfortable with yourself. Once your posture is perfect, the energy will flow and create miracles.

In all three parts of this kriya you lock your Mercury and Sun fingers down with your thumb. Use the thumb (which represents the id) to strongly press down the two fingers. The Jupiter and Saturn fingers point straight like antennae. In this mudra you control your communication and life flow with your identity, while you extend your wisdom and purity. Your eyes are closed and look down at the lunar center of the chin through the closed lids.

1. Sit in Easy Pose with a straight spine. Bend your elbows and press your upper arms against your ribcage. The forearms point upward. Your hands are in the mudra at shoulder level with the wrists bent and the palms facing upward. The Jupiter and Saturn fingers point to the sides with an upward angle of about sixty degrees. (The correct hand position will be uncomfortable, but do your best to keep the correct angle.) Keep your chin in, chest out, and your neck straight. Be steady to allow the energy to flow. 12 Minutes.

2. The mudra and focus of the eyes remain the same. Stretch your arms out to the sides and up at a 60 degree angle. Your arms are straight with no bend in either elbow or wrist. Sit calmly, quietly, peacefully. You will now absorb the energy you created in the first segment of the meditation. 3 Minutes.

3. Create a halo for yourself by bringing your arms over your head with the Jupiter and Saturn fingers of one hand touching the Jupiter and Saturn fingers of the other hand, palms facing down. Your hands are still in the mudra and no other part of the hands touch. Every muscle and molecule in your body shall be automatically energized. Enjoy the touch of the fingers. 1 1/2 Minutes.

To Finish: Inhale deeply, hold the breath for 15-20 seconds, while contracting every muscle and keeping the Jupiter and Saturn fingers of the two hands touching. Exhale. Repeat this sequence two more times and relax.

The Jupiter finger represents wisdom and knowledge. In the science of color therapy, its color is golden orange. The Saturn finger represents purity and its color is blue. The Sun finger represents the life flow and its color is bright red. The Mercury finger represents communication and its colors are green and white-green.

"Kundalini Yoga is uncoiling yourself to find your potential and your vitality and to reach for your virtues. There is nothing from outside. Try to understand that. All is in you. You are the storehouse of your totality." YB

34

March 27, 1995

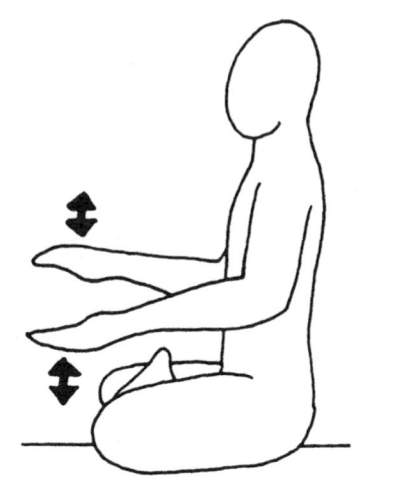

1. Sit in Easy Pose with your elbows bent and your upper arms near your rib cage. Your forearms point straight out in front of your body, parallel to the floor. The right palm faces downward and the left palm faces upward. Breathing through your nose, inhale in eight strokes and exhale in eight strokes. On each stroke of the breath, alternately move your hands up and down. One hand moves up as the other hand moves down. The movement of the hands is slight, approximately 6-8 inches, as if you are bouncing a ball. Breathe powerfully. Continue for 3 Minutes and then change the hand position so that the left palm faces downward and the right palm faces upward. Continue for another 3 Minutes and then change the hand position again so that the right palm faces downward and the left palm faces upward. Continue for a final 3 Minutes. (Total time for this first part of the meditation is 9 Minutes.)

"It doesn't matter if you know everything. The question is: do you practice?"
YB

2. Begin long, slow, deep breathing, stopping the movement and holding the position. Close your eyes and focus at the center of your chin. Keep your body perfectly still so it can heal itself. Keep your mind quiet, stilling your thoughts. 5 1/2 Minutes.

To finish: Inhale deeply, hold your breath, make your hands into fists and press them strongly against your chest. 15 Seconds. Exhale. Inhale deeply, hold your breath, and press your fists against your navel point. 15 Seconds. Exhale. Inhale deeply, hold your breath, bend your elbows bringing your fists near your shoulders and press your arms strongly against your rib cage. 15 Seconds. Exhale and relax.

This exercise balances the diaphragm and fights brain fatigue. It renews the blood supply to the brain and moves the serum in the spine. It also benefits the liver, navel point, spleen and lymphatic system.

The Healing Energies of the Earth and the Ether

May 9, 1995

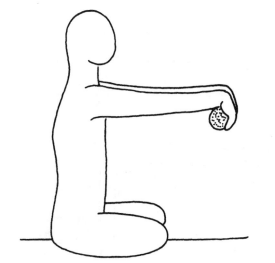

You will need an orange and a banana for this kriya. The orange represents the Ether and the banana represents the Earth.

1. Hold your arms straight out in front of your body at shoulder level. Allow your hands to hang down loosely from the wrists. Hold the orange in your right hand and the banana in your left hand, keeping the wrists absolutely loose. Your eyes are 9/10ths closed. Breathe in with eight strokes through your nose and breathe out with eight strokes through your mouth. Mentally chant "SA TA NA MA, SA TA NA MA" to count the strokes on each inhale and exhale. 11 Minutes.

To finish: Inhale deeply, hold the breath 15 seconds and stretch your arms straight out in front of you. Stretch from your shoulders. Exhale. Inhale deeply, hold the breath 15 seconds and stretch your arms straight up, stretching the spine. Exhale. Inhale deeply and bend your elbows, bringing your arms to your sides. Hold your breath 25 seconds as you squeeze your rib cage with your arms and elbows. Exhale and relax.

"When your body receives healing from you, this is the best healing."
YB

2. Eat your orange and banana mixed. Eat them both at the same time. Don't eat one and then eat the other.

After the first two and a half minutes of this meditation, you will enter a twilight zone in which you may feel pain all over your body. Keep breathing rhythmically and you can maintain yourself. The only thing that can save you from pain is the powerful breath. Nothing else. After five minutes your hands may start shaking, that is a normal reaction. Starting at seven minutes there may be a pressure on your spine for the next three minutes. Sit up straight and keep going. Don't tighten your wrists under any circumstance. When the spinal fluid starts changing and the body starts renewing itself, you may experience pain in the armpits. The armpits are where the brain releases its toxins. Keep breathing and go through it. For the last minute, breathe very heavily.

We use fruit in healing meditations because "Everything comes from out of the Word. Everything can be converted into purity of energy by the power of the Word." Banana lacks only citrus to be a complete food. By using a banana and an orange, we take a complete food, put in the energy of the power of the Word, and heal ourselves.

February 1, 1995

1. Sit in Easy Pose with a straight spine. Keep your chin in and your chest out. Raise your right arm straight up with the palm facing forward. Stretch your left arm straight out to the side parallel to the floor with the palm facing down. Split the fingers of each hand so that the Sun and Mercury fingers are together and the Jupiter and Saturn fingers are together. Close your eyes and meditate. 11 Minutes maximum.

"Reality is explainable."
YB

If you wish to use a mantra with this meditation, you may use "Har, Haray, Haree, Wahe Guru". You may chant it out loud, chant it mentally, or listen to a musical tape of the mantra. It is your choice.

To finish: Inhale deeply, hold your breath for 10 seconds, as you stretch your arms and tighten your entire body. Exhale and repeat this sequence 2 more times.

To practice this meditation for 40 days, alternate the arm position each day. The first day you practice with the right arm up and the left arm out to the side. The next day stretch the left arm up and the right arm out to the side and so on. (You must always keep your elbows straight.)

Your body will start healing itself after the first 2 minutes. The entire cellular system will interact to heal you. Your body shall start healing and every muscle shall start hurting. This posture will hurt as long as you have any toxins in your body. This is central nervous system control therapy. In exactly 11 minutes, your entire cellular system shall change.

After 40 days the meditation will start working on your subtle bodies. Whatever starts happening to you after 40 days, keep it to yourself. Don't speak of it to anyone.

This is the most powerful self-purification you can do. It can give you complete control of your being. It improves intuition and makes you powerful and healthy. You'll be free of all garbage: physical, mental, and spiritual.

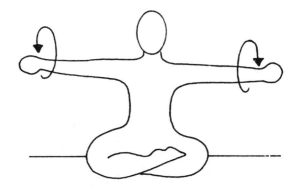

Regulate the Systems of the Body

August 31, 1995

1. Sit in Easy Pose with a straight spine. Stretch your arms out to the sides with the palms downward. On each hand, touch your thumb to the mound under the Mercury finger. Close your fist around your thumb. Keep your elbows straight as you revolve your arms and fists in backward circles that are 18" in diameter. The circles must be 18" wide for this movement to be effective. Breathe like a cobra, with a hissing breath <u>through the nose.</u>

Move quickly. The tape *Tantric Har* by Simran Kaur has the proper rhythm and can be used with this meditation. 11 Minutes.

To finish: Inhale, deeply fill the rib cage with air, hold the breath for 8 seconds and exhale powerfully, like cannon fire. Repeat this sequence two more times.

This meditation, done with the thumb touching the mound of Mercury, will communicate to every organ of the body to re-organize and regulate itself. It is calming and, if practiced for 120 days, will put everything in the body in rhythm. It can help menopause problems, glandular system problems, and regulate any part of the body that needs regulation.

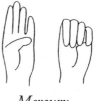

Mercury

Variations on this meditation:

• If you change the position of the thumb and keep all other aspects of the meditation the same, you can achieve different results.

Sun

• If the thumb is on the mound of the Sun finger, this meditation will give you energy and will fight disease.

• If the thumb is on the mound of the Saturn finger, it will give you purity and the experience of ecstasy.

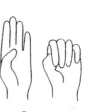

Saturn

• If the thumb is on the mound of the Jupiter finger, it will give you wisdom. In this mudra the Jupiter finger is extended, with the thumb touching the side of the Jupiter finger and all the other fingers closed as in the previous mudras.

These techniques are an effective way to get knowledge from the Unknown.

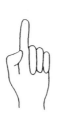

Jupiter

"Yoga was made for man to be healthy, happy and holy. Kundalini yuga was made for man to be healthy, happy, holy and aware. Secret of your soul is awareness."

"May I tell you something? There is only one thing you should know. Conquer yourself." YB

38

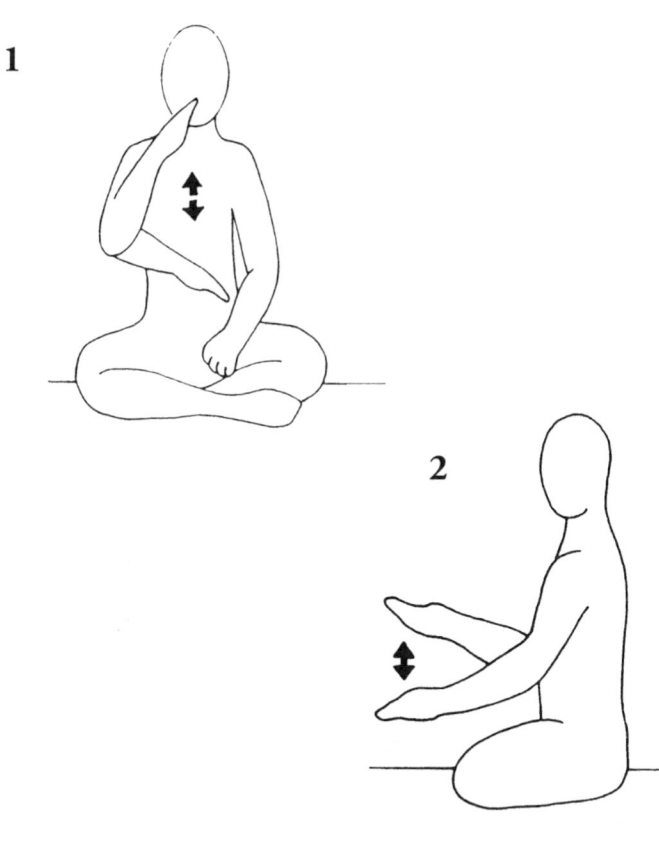

June 7, 1994

A Nine Minute Meditation to recover from the stress of life.

1. Bend your right elbow so that your forearm is in front of your body with the palm facing down. Without bending your wrist, move your right hand quickly up and down from the tip of your nose to your navel. Move fast and forcefully. Put your entire life force into the movement. Close your eyes and look at the center of your chin through your closed eyes. After 1 Minute make a tight fist of the left hand as you continue moving the right hand up and down for 2 Minutes more. This action affects the psyche of the heart.

"The techniques of Kundalini Yoga are an effective way to get knowledge from the Unknown." YB

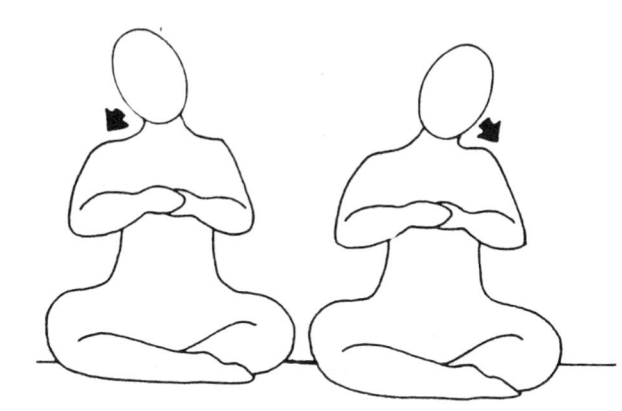

2. Sit with your arms down at your sides. Bend your elbows so that your forearms are parallel to the ground. The left palm faces downward towards the earth and the right palm faces upward toward the heavens. Alternately move each forearm up and down as if you were bouncing balls with your hands. Move powerfully. 3 Minutes. You are activating the earthly and heavenly elements within you at your own command and balancing them. (The pace is 1 to 3 movements per second.)

3. Place your hands at your heart center with the right hand over the left. Bend your neck to the left, bringing your left ear toward your left shoulder. Straighten your neck and bend your neck to the right, bringing your right ear toward your right shoulder. Continue leaning the head left and right. Close your eyes and mellow down into it. 2 Minutes. This exercise lets the neck adjust itself. Move smoothly into the next position without a break.

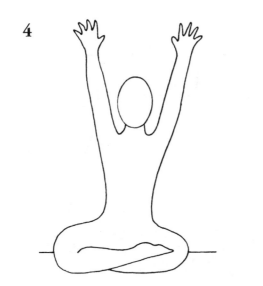

4

4. Stretch your arms straight up with the fingers open as wide as possible. Squeeze all the muscles in your body as you stretch upward. 1 Minute. Relax.

Stress is an essential part of modern life. Everyone needs techniques to de-stress themselves. This 9 minute meditation is a self-administered glandular control. The glands are the guardians of your health. You can trigger your own system to serve yourself. For example, in the first exercise, Yogi Bhajan says "the right hand sends a message of calm, while the left fist sends a message to the nervous system to wake up. The nervous system alerts the glandular system, the white corpuscles, and the cells. These two messages go to the brain which acts to balance the situation. The brain tells the pituitary, the master gland, to act. The pituitary tells the glandular system to do its best, the body works to come to balance, and the body chemistry will change."

June 19, 1996

1

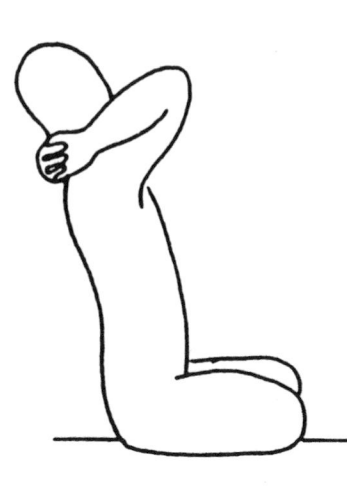

2

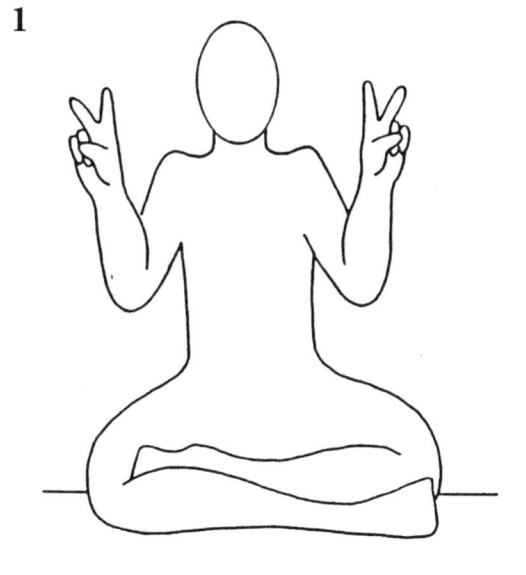

1. Sit in Easy Pose with your upper arms close to your sides. Your elbows are bent, your forearms extend upward, and your palms face forward. Your thumb locks the Mercury and Sun fingers. The Jupiter and Saturn fingers are split in a "V." Squeeze your shoulder blades together, which will push your rib cage one-half to one and one-half inches forward. Every muscle should be steel tight. Keep your chin pulled slightly in and your eyes closed. This meditation is done to the instrumental version of *Ardas Bhaee* on the tape called *Healing Sounds of the Ancients #5.* For 1 minute, whistle along with the tune. Then, for the next 2 minutes, chant the Ardas Bhaee mantra out loud from the navel. Really pull the navel in as you chant.

Ardas Bhaee, Amar Das Guru

Amar Das Guru, Ardas Bhaee

Ram Das Guru, Ram Das Guru

Ram Das Guru, Sachee Sahee

To finish: Lock your hands behind your neck and lean back sixty degrees. Inhale deeply and hold your breath for 10 seconds as you strongly pull the navel in. Exhale like cannon fire. Repeat this sequence two more times and relax.

"Meditation is the creative control of self where the Infinite can talk to you."
YB

To See the Unseen

April 7, 1994

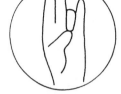

Left hand mudra

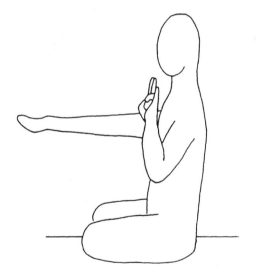

1. Sit in Easy Pose with your spine straight. Bend your left elbow so that your upper arm is near your ribs and the forearm and hand point upward. Your left palm faces forward in Surya Mudra, with the thumb and Sun finger touching. The other fingers point straight up. Stretch your right arm out in front of you with the palm cupped, facing upward, as if you are catching rainwater. There is no bend in the elbow. Close your eyes and focus at the center of your chin. Breathe slowly, consciously and deeply. 11 Minutes.

To finish: Inhale, hold your breath 15-20 seconds, as you stretch your right arm forward and squeeze every muscle in your body. Exhale like cannon fire. Repeat this sequence two more times. Relax.

2. Relax and take 5 Minutes to bring yourself back to normal consciousness. Talk, don't meditate.

Through this meditation the brain will create its own form of morphine to give the body endurance. The metabolism will change, the glands will secrete, the nervous system will be strengthened, and the brain will renew itself.

Do this meditation for 120 days straight, without a break, at the same time every day. Choose a particular time to do it each day so that you can establish a relationship between your automatic production of energy and the enhanced production of energy that this meditation enables your body to perform. You must establish a regular rhythm of practice. In time your automatic system will harmonize and take on the enhanced performance established by the meditation. It will change your metabolism. You will tune up your glandular system. "You will see the Unseen, a little bit. You will hear the Unheard, a little bit. You will know the Unknown, a little bit. You'll get a taste of it and you'll keep going."

To get a triple effect of this meditation, add two things to the above instructions. Roll your tongue backward against your upper palate and mentally chant "Wahe Guru". If you practice in this manner you _must_ have someone around to check on you and make sure you don't get lost in the meditation.

"Develop your intuition so that the changes in the years to come may be convenient for you." YB

42

Subagh Kriya

June 21, 1996

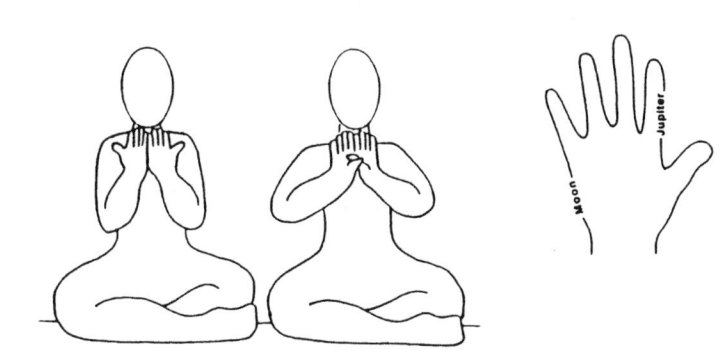

This is a 5 part kriya. Each part must be practiced for an equal amount of time, either 3 Minutes or 11 Minutes. Do not exceed 11 Minutes. Only the first exercise of this kriya may be practiced on its own, separately from the other exercises.

1. Sit in Easy Pose with a straight spine. Allow your upper arms to be relaxed, with the elbows bent and the palms in front of the chest. Strike the outer sides of the hands together, forcefully hitting the area from the base of the little finger (Mercury finger) to the base of the palm. This area is called the Moon area. Next strike the sides of the index fingers (Jupiter fingers) together. Hit hard! Alternately strike the Moon area and the Jupiter area as you chant "Har" with the tip of your tongue, pulling the navel with each "Har". Your eyes are focused at the tip of your nose. This meditation was taught to the rhythm of *Tantric Har* by Simran Kaur.

" I'm going to give you a very handy tool, one that you can use anywhere, and you'll become rich. To become rich and prosperous, with wealth and values, is to have the strength to come through. It means that transmissions from your brain and the power of your intuition can immediately tell you what to do." YB

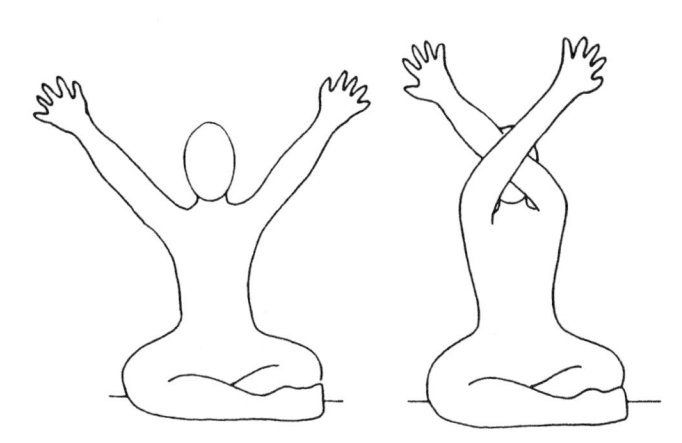

2. Stretch your arms out to the sides and up at a sixty degree angle. Spread your fingers wide, making them stiff. The palms face forward. Cross your arms in front of your face. Alternate the position of the arms as they cross: first the left arm crosses in front of the right and then the right arm crosses in front of the left. Continue crossing the arms, keeping the elbows straight and the fingers open and stiff. This movement is also done to the rhythm of *Tantric Har* by Simran Kaur, but this time you do not chant with the tape.

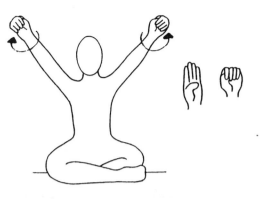

3

3. Keep your arms out and up at sixty degrees as in the previous exercise. With your hands, make a fist around your thumb, squeezing your thumb tightly as if you are trying to squeeze all the blood out of it. Move your arms in small backward circles as you continue squeezing your thumb. Your arms are stretched and the elbows stay straight. Chant the mantra "God" powerfully from your navel. One backward circle of the arms equals one repetition of "God." The speed and rhythm of the chanting is the same as in the previous exercises. Move powerfully so that your entire spine shakes, you may even be lifted slightly up off the ground by the movement.

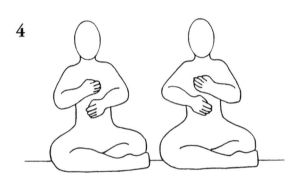

4

4. Bend your arms so that your elbows point to the sides. The forearms are parallel to the floor and the palms face the body around the level of the diaphragm. The right hand moves up a few inches as the left hand moves down. The left hand moves up as the right hand moves down. The hands move alternately up and down between the heart and navel. As the hands move, chant *Har Haray Haree, Whahay Guru* in a deep monotone with one repetition of the mantra approximately every 4 seconds. Chant from your navel. If you are practicing the exercises for 11 minutes each, then you will chant the mantra out loud for 6 Minutes, whisper it strongly for 3 Minutes, and then whistle it for 2 Minutes. If you are practicing the exercises for 3 minutes each, then you will chant the mantra out loud for 1 Minute, whisper it strongly for 1 Minute, and then whistle it for 1 Minute.

5

5. Bend your elbows and rest your right forearm on your left forearm, with your palms down. The arms are held in front of your body at shoulder height. Close your eyes, keep your arms steady. Keep your spine straight and your arms parallel to the floor. Breathe slowly and deeply so that one breath takes a full minute. Inhale for 20 seconds, hold for 20 seconds, and exhale for 20 seconds.

About Subagh Kriya, Yogi Bhajan has said "It's a complete set. This is all called Subagh Kriya. If God has written with His own hands that you shall live under misfortune, then by doing Subagh Kriya you can turn your misfortune into prosperity, fortune, and good luck."

November 13, 1985

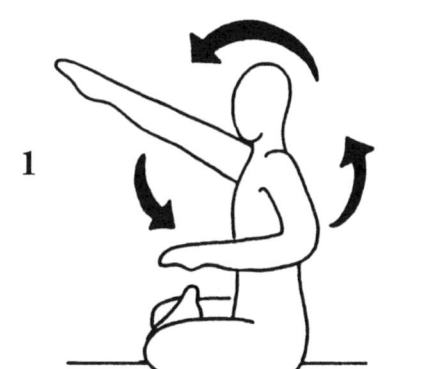

1

2

1. Sit in Easy Pose with your spine straight. Close your eyes. Move your arms as if you are swimming. Extend one and then the other in a constant motion. As you swim imagine yourself in a vast ocean as night is falling and a storm is coming. You can't see the shore, so use your intuition to determine which way to go to reach the shore. Whichever direction your intuition directs you, project yourself in that direction. Imagine that your survival depends on swimming in the right direction. Swim vigorously so the motion will automatically give you a special breath rhythm. 11 1/2 Minutes.

Only with a vigorous effort can you achieve the correct breath rhythm. Once you have achieved the breath rhythm then this creative pranayam will help you develop your ability to think intuitively.

2. Come into Baby Pose with the spine totally relaxed. As your head touches the floor imagine your relief that you have made it safely to the shore. Feel gratitude in every cell. 7 Minutes.

To finish: Inhale deeply and, while still in Baby Pose, move the spine in all directions to loosen it up. Let the spine readjust itself. Gradually rise up and relax.

"Intuitive projection and intuitive reception have the strength of guarding you. In America, the only appropriate way to describe it is they are your guardian angels." YB

Teachers open the door, but you must enter by yourself.

Chinese proverb

<u>Dhan Dhan Ram Das Gur</u>
Dhan Dhan Raam Daas Gur, jin siria tineh savaariaa
Poore hoee karamaat, aap siranjana-haareah dhaariaa
Sikhee ateh sangatee, paarabrahm kar namaskaariaa
Ata ataao atol too,tayraa ant na paaravaariaa
Jinee too sayviaa bhao kar, say tudh paar utaaria
Labh lobh kaam krodh moho, maar kadhe tudh saparavaariaa
Dhan so tayraa taan heh, sach tayraa pehsakaariaa
Nanak too lehenaa too heh, Gur Amar too veecharria
Guru ditta taa man saadhaariaa

Blessed, blessed is Guru Ram Das.
The Lord who created Thee, He alone has adorned Thee.
Complete is Thy miracle.
The Creator Himself has installed Thee on the throne.
Deeming Thee as the Transcendent Lord, Thine followers and congregations bow before Thee.
Thou art immovable, unfathomable, and immeasurable.
Thou hast no end or bounds.
They who serve Thee with love,
Them Thou ferriest across.
Avarice, covetousness, sexual desire, wrath and worldly love,
Thou hast beaten and driven out with all their ramifications.
Praiseworthy is Thy place,
True are Thine bounties.
Thou art Nanak, Thou art Angad,
Thou art Guru Amar Das, so do I deem Thee.
When I saw the Guru, then was my soul sustained.

Chattar Chakkar Vartee
Jaap Sahib: The Last Four Lines

Chattar chakkar vartee, chattar chakkar bhugatay
Suyumbhav subhang, sarab daa sarab jugatay
Dukaalang pranaasee, dayaalang saroopay
Sadaa Ang Sangay, abhangang bibhootay.

Thou art pervading in all the four quarters of the universe,
Thou are the enjoyer in all the four quarters of the universe.
Thou art self-illumined and united with all.
Destroyer of bad times, embodiment of mercy.
Thou art ever within us.
Thou art the everlasting giver of undestroyable power.

Ardas Bhaee

Ardas Bhaee, Amar Das Guru
Amar Das Guru, Ardas Bhaee
Ram Das Guru, Ram Das Guru
Ram Das Guru, Sachee Sahee

The prayer has been made to Guru Amar Das.
Guru Ram Das is the true guarantee the prayer has been.

Aad sach, jugaad sach, haibhay sach, Nanak hosee bhay sach

True in the beginning, true throughout the ages, Nanak the Infinite shall ever be true.

Har, Haray, Haree, Wahe Guru

The One, the Projected One, the Merged One, the Ecstacy of God.

Sat Nam

Truth is the identity of God

48

Sa Ta Na Ma

Infinity, birth, death, re-birth.

Mukande

God as Liberator

Hum Dham, Har Har

We are the Universe brought to the earth,
We are exalted to. God.

On the pronunciation of the mantra "Har"

The "a" in the mantra "Har" is pronounced like the "u" in "hug". The "r" is produced in a special way with just the tip of the tongue touching the roof of the mouth, behind the front teeth, to make the "r" sound.

The mantra is chanted by pulling the navel in strongly and, as the air is forced from the lungs, the sound "Har" flows out with the breath, ending as the tip of the tongue touches the roof of the mouth.

Tapes of these mantras and songs may be obtained from:
Golden Temple Enterprises
Box 13 Shady Lane
Espanola, NM 87532
Toll Free: 800-829-3970

Additional Copies of this manual may be obtained from:
Ancient Healing Ways
P.O. Box 130
Espanola, NM 87532
800-359-2940

NOTES